THE
ACTIVATED
WORD

ADRIEL NICOLE SPARKS

Unless otherwise noted, Scripture quotations are taken from the New King James Version.® Copyright © 1982 by Thomas Nelson, Inc. Used by permission. All rights reserved.

Scripture quotations marked NIV are taken from the Holy Bible, New International Version®. niv®. Copyright © 1973, 1978, 1984, 2011 by Biblica, Inc.™ Used by permission. All rights reserved.

Scripture quotations marked MSG are taken from THE MESSAGE. Copyright © by Eugene Patterson 1993, 1994, 1995, 1996, 2000, 2001, 2002. Used by permission of NavPress Publishing Group. All rights reserved.

Printed in the United States of America

Published in Hellertown, PA

Library of Congress Control Number:

2021910080

ISBN: 978-1-952481-23-9

2 4 6 8 10 9 7 5 3 1 paperback

Book cover and interior design by Adriel Nicole Sparks

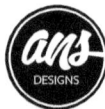

www.adrielnicolesparks.com

He sees something special in you.
Let's find out what that is...

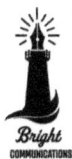

Bright Communications LLC

Hellertown, PA

My Heart

To my Father,
Lord, I want to thank You for using me to write
something so dear to my heart. As long as You are
pleased, the toil has paid off. I love You beyond
measure.

To my husband and best friend,
Baby, you are my rock. There is no place I'd rather
be than here in this marriage with you.
Let's do life, forever.

To my children,
The three of you are my greatest gifts. Individually,
you are anointed vessels of God. Together, you are a
force to be reckoned with. Don't ever break
that bond.

THE PACKAGE

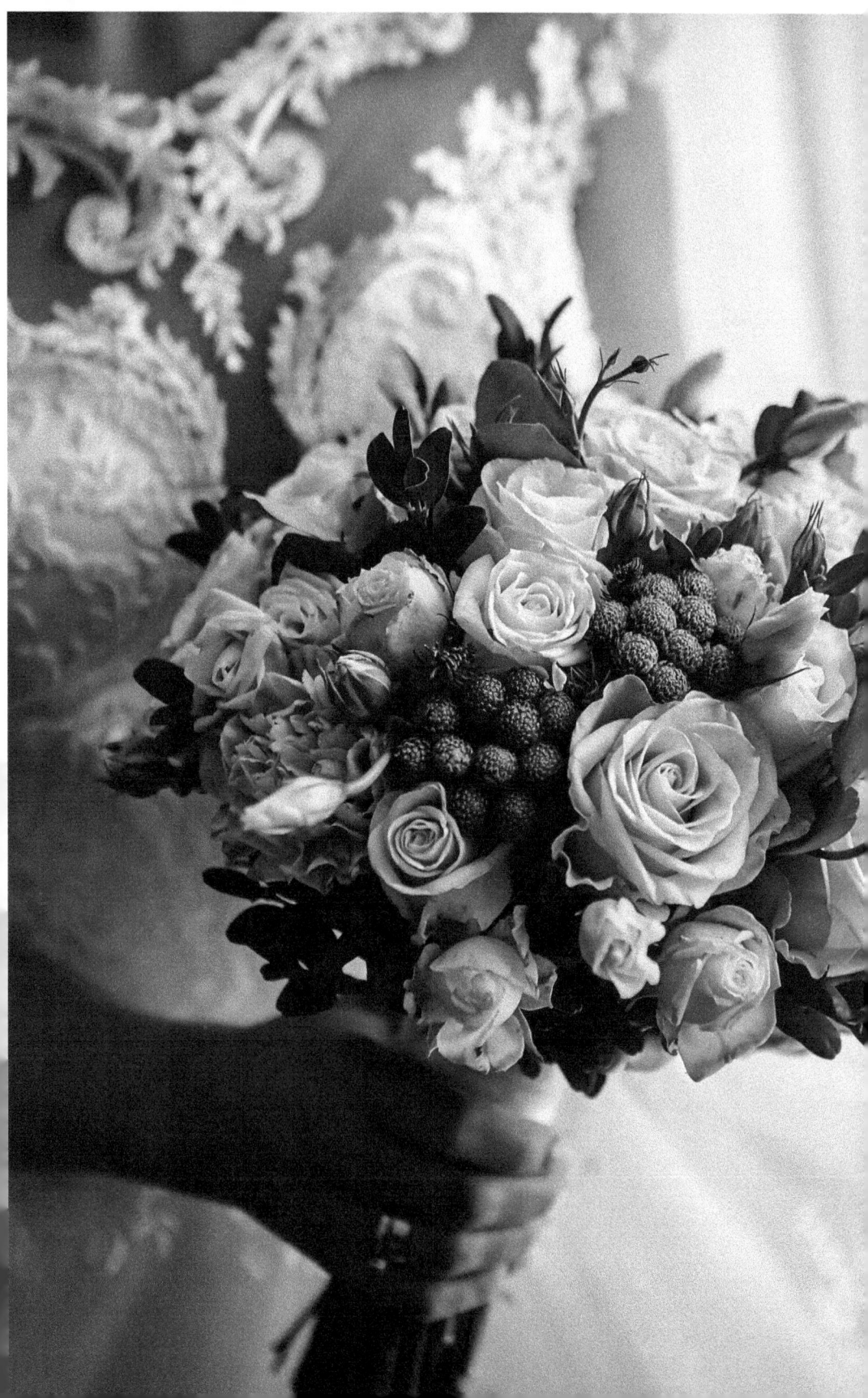

INTRODUCTION

'TIL DEATH DO US PART

"Depression is not defined by race, gender, age, background history, or level of attraction. It should not be a checklist of things you need to fill out for someone to take you seriously. We may not sob in public, but that doesn't mean it's not killing us on the inside. Depression is a camouflaged titan, and the person living with it surely has a fight on their hands."

If that quote resonated with you, I assume you and depression have met before. Perhaps he's stolen your fight. Perhaps you've been emptied. I need to let you know that you are not alone. I've been there. My name is Adriel, and I'm a wife and mother who has faced years of mental damage. Both depression and anxiety placed their bets on my death.

Having dealt with the afflictions for so long, I started referring to them as people disguised as blood-sucking leeches. The three of us had a *'til death do us part* type of bond. A twisted polygamy. This abusive relationship became a lifestyle that I was sure I would never recover from. Weeping until pieces of my skin could almost break off from dry tears was normal for me. Sorrow was the pillow that I slept with after sunset. My insecurities were the curtains that I opened before the sun rose.

Now, this wasn't a rapid spread. Nor was it easily detected. For a while, I thought I was just stressed. My depression started out as a few moments of sadness, then progressed to mood swings. It reduced my self-esteem, and finally, I lost functioning in my brain and body. I transformed into an empty cloud of smoke sitting at the gates of death. My life became lifeless, and a lingering spirit of darkness swallowed me whole. I cursed the day God chose me as His alleged perfect creation. Suicide wrapped its hands around my neck and strangled me.

The ache of wanting to die but feeling terrified of Hell remains fresh in my mind. It's a feeling you never really forget. I remember standing in my kitchen one day, deciding whether I should develop a cutting habit. I had grown numb to every emotion that I was desperate enough to physically hurt myself. Cutting was something that I saw the depressed take for a spin, making me eager to try it all the more. I hunted for the sharpest knife in the drawer and attempted the first cut. Raising the blade above my left wrist and diving into the lateral side of it, I looked to slice away the wrath. However, no ounce of blood was shed. The only thing left was a line of ash where the knife should have penetrated my skin. I tried harder the second time around, and yet, not a single tinge of red.

When I began to try for a third time, my husband walked in and grabbed the knife, "Baby, what are you doing?"

I cried out, "Just let me do it. It's the only thing that'll make me feel human again! You don't understand what I'm up against!"

It took a minute for me to snap back into reality, for it all felt strange. All I could envision was how badly I wanted to self-harm. Life wasn't worth another second of this agony. I thought cutting would be a great way to deal with it, a temporary antidote. But my husband saw things differently. In a hurry to stop me, he gathered every knife he could find and hid them from my reach. I sank my head into the kitchen counter and cried until I entered a daze.

A similar episode came about after a heated discussion with him one afternoon. In this case, anger ingested me. It began to swell at my feet and climb to the top of my head. The threat was so intense that it welcomed a panic. I was discouraged in knowing that not even my spouse would take the time to consider that I was ill. He chuckled in bafflement when I tried to justify my illness, and it drove me mad. I remember thinking, *I'm abandoned by my family, stricken by my brain, and worst of all, forsaken by God Himself. What else is there for me to live for?*

Bitterness took over as these thoughts flooded my mind during the argument. Fire scorched my insides as I panted for air. There was only one solution left in that instant.

To create an escape plan.

To jump out of my skin, no matter what it took.

I jetted downstairs and headed toward our kitchen balcony, determined to leave misery behind that day. But what's that saying again? *Misery loves company?* While my plan to flee was standing seconds away, depression wanted me around for a bit longer. As I swung open the door, my husband yanked me backward and grappled with me until I became stable.

Just writing this brings tears to my eyes. The pain was surreal. I was trapped in a paralyzing nightmare that I could not awaken from. Suicide broadcasted louder than any reason to live, proving that I would never recover the old me.

Here's the kicker though: My story doesn't end in agony.

This story? This story ends in an abundance that sweats through my pores. Without a doubt, I French kissed the edge of fatality, though I later discovered a morsel of strength nudging through the fabric of my back pocket. That token of courage paid for God's grace. He embraced me into His arms and awakened my purpose. Now, He's granted me the opportunity to help you awaken yours.

This book is your personalized gift from the Creator. It's your "get out of death for freedom" card and your royal voucher into a renewed life of everlasting joy.

"

YOU CANNOT
FIGHT A THING
WITHOUT KNOWING

ITS DNA.

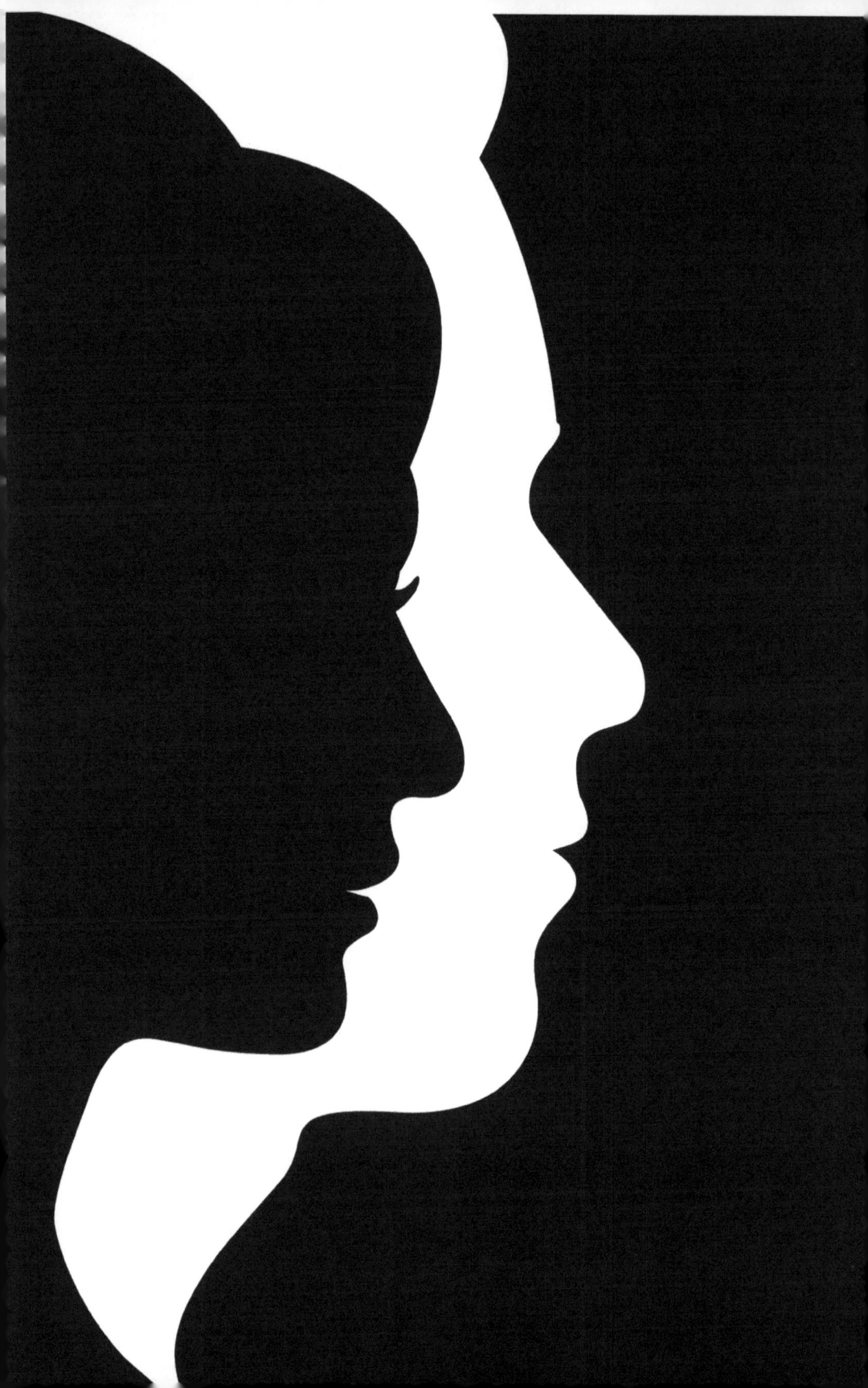

CHAPTER ONE

EXPOSING THE ENEMY

PART A

the leftovers

During my sufferance, all I hunted for was a tender ear. I wanted someone to know how grueling this was. I needed them to pop open a window for me to vent without dusty conditions or sly remarks. I rummaged for that space in people I fostered a lifetime of rapport. Yet I found not a soul willing to say, "Come." No one to accept solace from. No one to latch my grief on to. I felt deserted, as if my body was wounded and thrown into the ocean for sharks to salivate over. I began to question whether life itself had been authentic all this time.

Does the world even exist? Is God a fictional Character? Am I repeating the same day over again, or could this honestly be the meat of my being?

Life is supposed to be about happiness, love, peace, and chasing dreams. This wasn't the design of my luck. Not even close. I was breathing in carbon monoxide and exhaling the oxygen that necessitated my survival. I was death's mistress! I saw the world in shades of black and gray instead of the picturesque colors that my eyes once loved. I was a defective copy of a human, a fraud who failed to get tested by the Maker before gushing me out. I was the outcast. The decrepit fruit. The leftovers. Depression dug holes in my brain and tried to take me out. I was vulnerable, and he stripped me bare.

For this reason, I'm here to return the favor. With God's hand, I've murdered a vulture. I have overcome the greatest war of one's life—the battle of the mind. Therefore, it is my honor to wash away the concealer, lay it out raw, and expose the skeleton of depression.

PART B
the mental breakdown

I find it interesting what happens to the grimy waste that we toss into the dumpster each week. About 26% is burned to ashes;

44% is salvageable, and the outstanding 30% is broken down and chemically decomposed into smaller fragments.[1] Foods like pizza, chicken, and burgers become unrecognizable in a matter of days. All that remains is the chemical equation for their physical formation. What if I told you that the answers to cancer, diabetes, hypertension, heart disease, and the flu could be rooted in the breakdown of what you've left unnoticed? The secrets to your health are immersed in wisdom. If we scrutinized our food's chemical nature, mortality rates would lessen and our quality of life would rise.

That information holds slight value in the common eye, though.

Many of us would rather satisfy our palates than accept that knowledge is power—with health awareness being a critical element of our existence. *Power over pleasure* should be the notion of this planet. But sadly, it has never been that way. We will choose medication and healthcare visits over prevention any day. Society teaches us to cover everything up with a pharmaceutical veil, while they profit from our flesh using our most dependable substance: food. Physicians spend more time training in restoration than they do in nutritional literacy. And because we're absent-minded, accepting poison from this broken system becomes a habit we never seem to escape. They control us, and we let them.

Now let's replace the words "waste" and "society" with our chief focus. Like food, diseases of the mind are formed out of chemicals yet disguised as our thoughts. Depression fools us into believing all that we are not, and nothing that we certainly are.

But he nurses a more delicate nature than the mere excess of food. Mental waste is harder to classify than a physical ailment, such as a broken leg or type 2 diabetes. A condition like diabetes is pretty straightforward. The body either doesn't produce enough insulin, or it opposes the insulin being produced. This leaves the prognosis to be fairly simple; diet and exercise can normally manage the symptoms. If it fails, insulin therapy or medication will suffice.

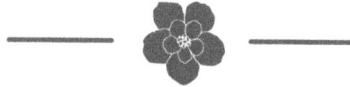

———— ✿ ————

When you look up the standard definition of depression, it's not as helpful. You'll likely see something like this:

Depression is characterized by feelings of severe despondency and dejection.[2]

If you search a little further, you may get this:

Depression (Major Depressive Disorder) is a common and serious medical illness that negatively affects how you feel, how you think, and how you act. Depression causes feelings of sadness and loss of interest in activities once enjoyed. It can lead to a variety of emotional and physical problems, and can decrease a person's ability to function at work and at home.[3]

The problem with these definitions is that they negate a fundamental concept: the science behind the disorder. They magnify the victim's emotions, rather than the chemistry of the invader. That's why treatment involves seeing a psychiatrist or a counselor to discuss your low-spirited "feelings." How can we settle for that? This condition is greater than just your temperament. We're talking about the faltering of one of the most crucial organs of the human body, the brain.

I needed to study the makeup of depression to get real answers. What is it exactly? Where does it come from? How is it formed? I wanted to unmask its core. You cannot fight a thing without knowing its DNA. That's like Mayweather preparing for a boxing match without having learned his opponent first. You think he'd win? Probably not. The same applies here. Anytime God does something new in your life, He always exposes the old. He reveals what has taken guardianship over you to help you slay it. You basically get the cheat codes on how to break out of prison. In this arena, depression is your prison, and I'm handing over the keys to break you out. But first, I need to break down this sickness and refine its definition.

Depression is *best* defined as a disease in which neurotransmitters and various parts of the brain either underperform or overexert their functions.

Six neurotransmitters and regions of the brain are off balance in depression, including the following:

Norepinephrine (also called noradrenaline)

- Regulates mood and concentration
- In the depressed, norepinephrine levels are diminished—giving rise to mood swings, a loss of pleasure, and difficulty focusing (which places you at risk for ADHD).

Serotonin (also referred to as the "happy chemical")

- Regulates attention, mood, social behavior, appetite, digestion, sleep, memory, and arousal
- When you're depressed, serotonin levels are minimized—leading to an inability to express happiness, anxiety, poor memory, low self-esteem, difficulty sleeping, aggression, digestive issues, and a reduced libido.

Dopamine

- Affects learning, movement, attention, motivation, sleep, and pleasure
- Dopamine is lessened in depression—lowering your ability to retain information, decreasing your equilibrium (which may cause clumsiness), creating insomnia, reducing your energy, and declining pleasure in activities once enjoyed.

The Amygdala

- A part of the brain that is correlated with negative

emotions. It stimulates when a person gives off an undesirable response to a situation.

- The amygdala is hyperactive in depression, which triggers the production of stress hormones in the HPA axis. This increase in hormones inhibits the prefrontal cortex and affects memory and learning.

Atrophy of the Frontal Lobes and Hippocampus

- The frontal lobes of the brain manage emotional reactions, motor functions, memory, problem-solving, social behavior, and sexual performance.
- The hippocampus is responsible for memory and emotions. If it withers, it can lead to Alzheimer's disease.
- In depression, the frontal lobes and hippocampus shrink in size—also known as atrophy—which compromises knowledge retention and emotional and physical disposition.

Several areas of a depressed brain can be imbalanced around the same time, leaving the effects of each to have an even greater impact on your behavior. For example, both serotonin and norepinephrine regulate mood. When both transmitters decrease, the chances of the victim being happy is twice as low.

Depression is an ugly disease. I wouldn't wish it on my worst enemy. Imagine my regret when I realized that I had been sick with multiple forms of mental illness. If you're like me, you've also met a few of his family and friends. Anxiety, chronic depression, and perinatal depression all had it out for me. They wrapped me into a straitjacket and force-fed me their venom. As a result, I have also exposed them.

Chronic depression is a long-lasting form of depression that lingers for at least two years. The victim is nearly impossible to treat and may find difficulty maintaining daily activities.

Perinatal depression is a combination of antepartum and postpartum depression. It is a disease in which a dramatic change in hormones, such as estrogen and progesterone, affects a pregnant woman's central nervous system (CNS). Symptoms can appear at any time during the pregnancy, and they can last for several years if left untreated. Mothers experience intense sorrow, anxiety, insomnia, frustration, and exhaustion that make it tough for them to care for themselves and the baby. Depression before the pregnancy can raise these symptoms.

One in seven women will have some form of pregnancy-related depression, and women from all backgrounds are at risk for it, regardless of a healthy or unhealthy pregnancy, married or unmarried, first-time mother or not, planned or unplanned pregnancy, and irrespective of age, race, income, or education.[4]

Generalized anxiety is a disorder in which the neuroanatomical functions of the brain become hyperactive. A person may show signs of angst, rapid breathing, increased heart rate, irritability, verbal stammering, restlessness (or feeling on edge), unexplained fear, brain fog, muscle tension, fatigue, and sleep disturbance. People who also deal with **social anxiety** may avoid others for fear of being embarrassed by two kinds of attacks:

1. **Panic attacks.** These happen suddenly, and they involve overwhelming fear. Symptoms include rapid heart rate, shortness of breath, nausea, fear of dying or losing control, trembling, tightness in throat, dizziness, or headache. These attacks are usually brought on by external stressors and can happen whether a person feels calm or anxious. They generally last between a few minutes to an hour.

2. **Anxiety attacks.** These are buildable, inner emotional rages that appear to be caused by fear of a problem that may surface. Although this is similar to panic attacks (i.e. a racing heartbeat, a knot in the stomach, etc.), these are less severe. However, both can occur at once; and they often do in people with depression and anxiety.

Before moving any further, let's recap what we've just learned. Here are symptoms that people with these afflictions may suffer from. They range from mild to severe, and severity depends on the length of exposure. They include:

- Sorrow
- Low self-esteem
- Loss of interest or pleasure in activities once enjoyed
- Changes in appetite
- Trouble sleeping or sleeping too much

- Loss of energy
- Psychomotor impairment
- Slowed speech or stammering
- Difficulty thinking, concentrating, and making decisions
- Suicidal thoughts
- Decline in memory
- Loss of sex drive
- Increased irritability and aggression
- Rapid breathing or heart rate
- Restlessness
- Fear of social interaction

What causes depression to settle in the brain?

Depression can breed from six different factors: trauma, stress, sustaining medical problems, hormonal imbalance, nutritional deficiencies, and simply trying to find your identity. Because chemicals in the CNS define mood disorders, any abnormality in the body will make it conducive for mental illness.

Five Insane Facts about Depression:[5]

1. More than 264 million people of all ages suffer from depression worldwide.
2. Globally, depression is the leading cause of disability, and it is also a major contributor to the overall burden of disease.
3. If left untreated, depression can lead to suicide.
4. Nearly one half of those who battle depression also

have an anxiety disorder.

5. Women experience depression two times the rate of men, and here's why:

    - **Those crazy hormones!** Estrogen and progesterone are amplified in women, which can cause a hormonal imbalance.

    - **Who does society say I am?** As young girls, we're trained to be sensitive to how the world sees us. *Act like a lady* is a phrase we've heard too often, and it makes us obsess over our looks and behavior. The focus is placed on "Will they approve of me?" instead of "How do I envision myself?" These ultimatums throw us into the trunk of a car operated by false identity for most of our lives, and in the end, we're caught in a slump—never knowing who we really are. On the other hand, men are raised to be autonomous and absent of emotion. The phrase *act like a man* is said more often to them than the words "I love you," so they have a harder time soaking in their feelings.

    - **Our brains are wired differently.** Women lack the biological gift to forget any situation that has broken their hearts. Because of gender differences in the amygdala, we retain more vivid memories than males. Naturally, men access the right side of this structure—which reduces thought and detail but calls for a physical response. This is why men are seen punching holes in the wall when they're upset. Women are just the opposite, though. We neglect the right in favor of the left. That's why we're seen crying or raising our voices when we're hurt.

- **Stress.** On average, women experience more stressful events in childhood that prevent us from coping as adults. Childhood abuse, for example, is more common in the female gender.

- **Suicidal media.** We exist in the 21st century, where many of us are governed by our phones. People can't even drive without their faces being plastered to a newsfeed. We convert as media addicts, and it kills our mentality. In fact, a social media and depression study performed on young adults in 2017 was quite discouraging. The outcome stated that the suicide rate in the female gender has risen by more than 65% since the late 2000s.[6] That number should come as no surprise, considering Myspace originated in 2003, Facebook and Twitter were founded in 2004, YouTube sprouted in 2005, Instagram arrived in 2010, and Snapchat hit in 2011.

Whether or not we choose to admit it, we all compare ourselves to those on social media. Positions of beauty, lifestyle, careers, and fame are deemed the most important things to achieve or you're not actually living. Rates of body dysmorphia and eating disorders have also risen because of this. When a woman realizes she cannot live up to those standards, her self-love begins to spiral into self-hate, and suicide is often the result.

The Sad Truth About Suicide:[7]

- Nearly 800,000 people in the world commit suicide per year—that equates to one life lost every 40 seconds.
- Depression is the leading cause of suicide, and suicide is the second leading cause of death in 15-29-year-olds.
- Females attempt suicide three times as often as males, and poisoning is the most common method of self-slaughter.

Here's what you should know about antidepressants.

One out of ten people over the age of 12 is prescribed antidepressants per year.[8] That percentage is horrible, given that after months of being on the treatment, symptoms can return into a full-blown relapse. This setback demands the physician to either increase the dosage or place the patient on a much stronger medication. But they fail to grasp that the brain is considering the antidepressants to be foreign. So, the drugs are more harmful than they are helpful.

The majority of antidepressants, such as SSRIs, work by

preventing your body from reabsorbing serotonin. This causes an excess amount of serotonin to circulate in the area outside of the neurons. The drugs are trying to stabilize the brain by doing this, but really, they're just allowing things to swim where they don't belong. And in the end, symptoms continue to show up because the brain does not approve of an illusionary balance.

People remain on this medication for years, leaving the effects of these drugs to be life-threatening instead of life-saving.

10 Reasons to Say NO to Antidepressants:[9]

1. Studies show that the percentage of people who claim to experience a relief of symptoms is nearly equal to the number of people given a placebo, which is just a sugar pill. Hence, there is rare proof that they work.
2. There's a high risk of relapse when you stop taking the medication.
3. Antidepressants can lead to Parkinson's disease and tardive dyskinesia.
4. They can kill the neurons in the brain, leading to a worse cognitive decline.
5. They may increase the risk of breast cancer.
6. Gastrointestinal functioning is often impaired while on this medication.
7. Sexual dysfunction can be further reduced.
8. They are associated with child developmental issues, such as autism, if taken by a pregnant or lactating mother (to whom they're often prescribed).

9. There's a higher risk of abnormal bleeding and stroke while on antidepressants.
10. People over the age of 50 are at risk for falling, further memory loss, bone fracturing, hyponatremia, and even death.

Whew! Well, how about psychologists and therapists? Should I make an appointment to see one?

Short answer: I wouldn't recommend it. Depression is not wholly consumed with emotions. It originates in the green light system of the body, the CNS. Your emotional output is just a product of your brain's faulty input. Remember, it's a chemical imbalance. Therefore, seeing a counselor may not be the best option. Their job is to get you to expel your feelings while they listen out for keywords to prescribe you something. They play God in your life, giving you advice on situations they may have never gone through. You entrust them with your buried secrets, and you hardly know them. A psychologist will pick up the pieces that you've laid down and stick you in a class with everyone else as a "one size fits all." Let's be real, you're paying for a ripped bandage to adhere to a blood-gushing wound.

There is a third dimension to depression.

Up until this point, we have unlocked two realms: the psychological realm in which emotions are shown and the chemical nature beneath it. Though we've seen the bulk, let's dissect it a layer deeper. Depression is parallel to the human design. Humans are three-dimensional figures: We have a body (our connection to the world), a spirit (our connection to God), and a soul (our eternal lifeline). Depression is kind of the same. It has a body (which highlights its human makeup), a spirit (which connects us to a lie-line), and a soul (which connects us to the engineer of the lie-line). Who is the engineer in this case? Say hello to the author of confusion, the Enemy.

Scripture tells us that our struggle is not against what we can physically see, but against the unseen things. We are fighting the armies in the supernatural realm. Mental illness is a cold-blooded attack on the Body of Christ. If you can take out the mind, you can take out the entire Body. Satan has invented a way to control the minds of God's people. He is planning to behead you so you'll never obtain what is rightfully yours—freedom.

When God directed me for this chapter, He sorted out the depression terms into an acronym that caught my attention. The first letter of *serotonin, amygdala, tricyclic antidepressants, and norepinephrine* aligned into one five-letter word: SATAN.

SEROTONIN

AMYGDALA

TRICYCLIC

ANTIDEPRESSANTS

NOREPINEPRHINE

I was amazed when I wrote this down. The message could not have been any clearer. From the start, Satan has been the master manipulator behind the rewiring of our brains. Mental illness is the façade that he puts on to keep us from identifying him. He pours liquids of self-doubt and fear into our hearts. He urges practitioners to medicate us while sending our anatomy into turmoil. Satan wants us to breathe, eat, and vomit toxins. He wants to dupe you into believing that you are the bad seed. That way, you can't navigate his web of lies. Like a preying tarantula, the devil knows just how to trap you. Now, his plan is wise but it lacks authority.

This is our time to catch him in action, to open the power package that God has sent for us to break him in half.

My boldness has grown after being freed from the teeth of the Enemy. It's been a long time coming, too. I used to be sinking in quicksand. Everyone tattooed their judgments onto my thinned-out skin. People conjured up their advice and spat it in my direction. They duct-taped me to the wrong frame of mentality, making me appear as someone with pessimistic thinking, instead of someone in need of saving.

They saw it all wrong. This was bigger than my thoughts. Depression mentally held me captive and physically changed how my body functioned. Like most of you, I was seen as just another emotional woman left to battle this parasitical beast on my own. My goodness, even in our sickness, we're confronted with gender discrimination.

Women are so misunderstood, belittled, muted, and always told to change our attitude that we slide into a place of ineffective healing. Opinions get stuck in places they shouldn't be. But unless a person has seen the many faces of depression, they will never understand the battle of the mind.

ACT
on this!

Get out pen and paper, or use
whatever you have on hand,
and write down all of the ways
depression has ruined your life.
This is YOUR chance to expose
the enemy at the root and
behead his control over you.
Be as expressive as possible,
and don't hold back!

THE FURTHER WE LEARN,
THE STRONGER WE BECOME.
THE STURDIER WE ARE,
THE LOWER THE THREAT
OF ECHOED FRACTURE.

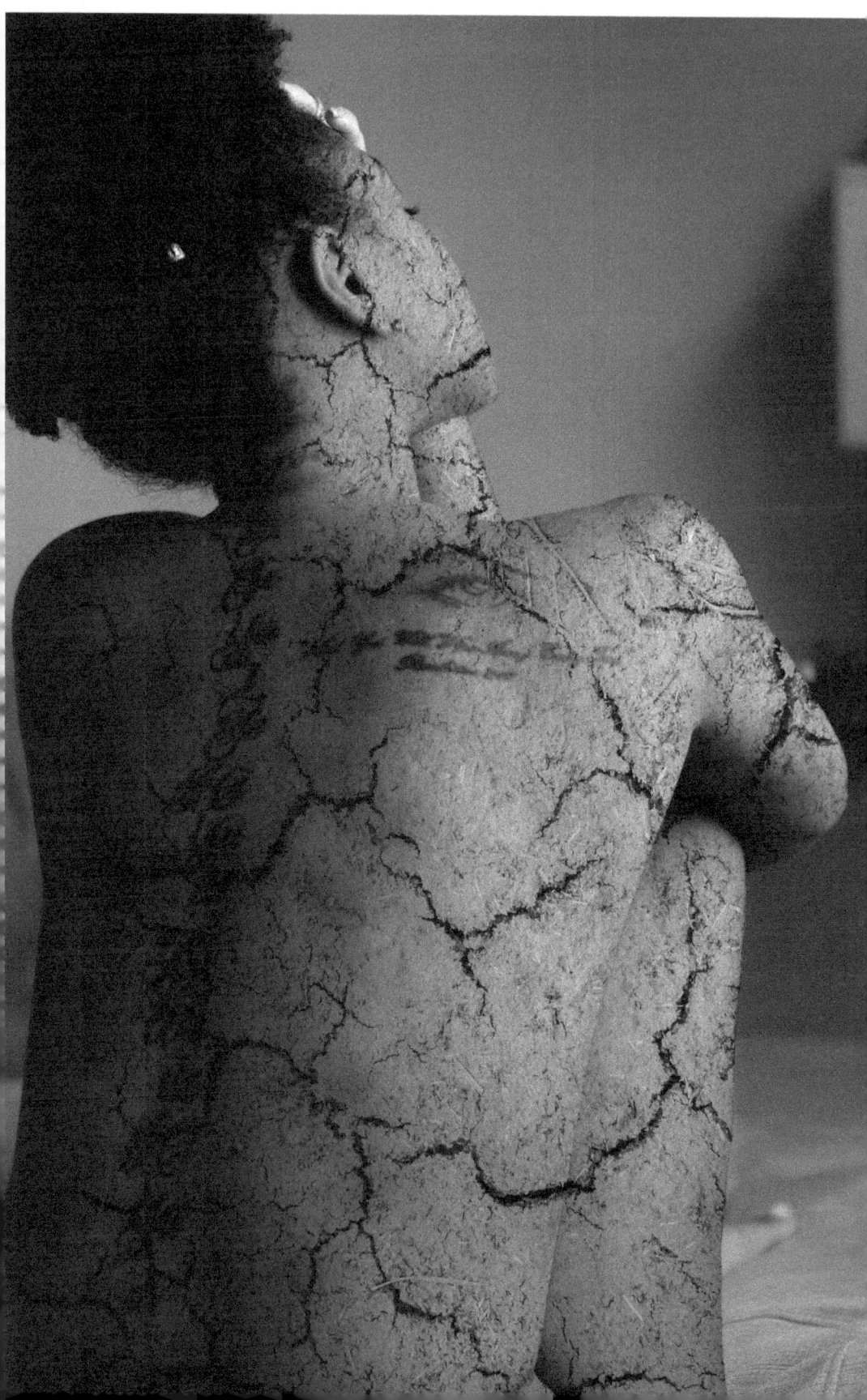

CHAPTER TWO

BROKEN CRAYONS

Being cultured in a religious home, I was a soft-hearted little girl who was friendly with everyone. You know the type: the pretty and bright princess that you see smiling from ear to ear. I suppose my cheerful attitude was based on my faith in the Gospel. My father left when I was two years old. His exit began a strong prayer life in my toddler years, and from then on, I used my playtime as God's time. Speaking the Word, laying hands, falling out in the Spirit, and singing and dancing to Christian music were childhood games that I loved. Pure and sweet was all I knew how to be. Tragically, that noble heart melted away, as self-conflict regarding my place in society became an enduring war.

A young lady from church invited me over when I was five. She was a close friend of ours and allowed me to sit with her during worship. The evening I went home with her, she molested me. The act was so intense that she took away my virginity. I struggled to explain to my mother what happened, and she later rushed me to the doctor's office. After careful examination of my body, the results confirmed that I had been molested. Or, in this case, raped. She'd successfully broken my hymen tissue—that which surrenders your innocence. The doctor warned my mother that my sensitivity had been heightened, and it would remain at that level for the rest of my life. The abuse paved a way for chronic lesbian activity, and it distorted my character. Before I knew anything, I was battling something I was too young to understand.

Many people are unaware of the damage that childhood trauma can cause. No one gives it the care it deserves because abuse is seen as something that just happens to people. They choose to patch it up and move on. But moving on keeps us in harm's way. Every 73 seconds, a person is sexually assaulted. Every nine minutes, that person is a child.[1] There are 58,400 children shattered by sexual abuse every year. The numbers continue to grow, and no one opens up about it. Fear, humiliation, and bewilderment keep us silent and repressed. You ever think that maybe this will continue to strike until we start speaking up? I'm a firm believer that telling your story could help save another.

So, today, I am a victim who is choosing to be loud. My past has silenced me for so long that I refuse to stay tongue-tied any longer. I'm sick of not getting to the root of my sorrow. We should be studying our scars, not hiding in shame. The further we learn, the stronger we become. The sturdier we are, the lower the threat of echoed fracture. It is only in your fight that you will change the future. Thus, I made a covenant with myself to find out how my past harm had affected me. It's also served as the connecting piece to my story.

I decided to research my trauma; and to my disbelief, the assault did more than I would have ever thought.

When you're sexually abused as a child, low self-esteem can make finding your identity an impossible mission. You face resistance when forming trustworthy relationships. Reaching a goal in life feels like sand escaping through your fingers. Managing stress plummets you to the point of crushing. Your sexual behavior leaves you to be tampered with. You are clothed in guilt, humiliation, anger, and self-blame. Nightmares taunt you until you're afraid to lie down at night. Brain development ceases, keeping you imprisoned to the age of the abuse. And finally, you surrender to addiction to help you gain back the tiniest bit of control. Assault is traumatizing. It sucks you into a creature that rules everything you say and every move you make. Victims from all over deal with it on their own because they cannot figure out how to communicate it.

"Will this person get it? Does it sound stupid to be stuck in my past? I can't even explain what's happened to me."

They aren't sure of how people will respond, so they stay mute. They are also prevented from learning more about what they're going through. Youth-focused trauma is experienced in several different waves of life. Still, we each have one common factor: We never get over the abuse. I was blind to the aftermath that shadowed my assault. It wasn't until I sat down and explored it fully that I was able to pinpoint what it did to me. I later saw that my whole future had been brutally shaped because of it.

Abuse at an early age can amplify the weight of the effects on victims, and they most often involve these outcomes:[2]

1. Psychological harm or hindrance of brain development—including behavioral issues, poor self-esteem, academic problems, and dysfunctional relationships
2. 80% of abused children are diagnosed with at least one psychiatric condition by the age of 21, such as anxiety, depression, eating disorders, or PTSD.
3. Studies show that abused children are 25% more likely to become pregnant before their 20th birthday.
4. Recurring thoughts of the assault—including nightmares or flashbacks
5. Difficulty raising their own children
6. Uncontrollable emotional reactions
7. Insomnia
8. Headaches
9. General victimization by others (i.e. childhood bullying)
10. Sexual disturbances of arousal, desire, or orgasm

11. Addiction to drugs, alcohol, sex, pornography, or masturbation

Victims may notice these effects immediately, in episodic flashes, or later on in life. There will be some kind of an attachment to their behavior. As said earlier, I had no idea how it overpowered me until I became an adult. Being a young girl without proper methods to heal, my brain tucked away the abuse. When your mind fails to sort out trauma, those memories are placed in the unconscious part of your brain. This process is known as dissociation. Your body will remember. Your conscious will not.

Nightmares from my childhood were the perfect example of a fight between the actual trauma and my amnesia. Though I couldn't remember the rape, it was stored in a mental compartment that would tear open and reveal itself in my dreams. I wandered off to sleep some nights and found myself in bed with a woman I did not recognize. Her face was unknown, but I believe she symbolized the rape as a whole. The lights were dimmed, the house remained quiet, and I would find myself detained to her bed. She'd walk toward me with a cunning smile on her face, and I could sense that something was off. I would also feel an unusual tingling in my genital area that was discomforting yet pleasing. She took me through a whirlwind of emotions that I should not have known about, and it scared me enough to try and leave the dream. But when I attempted to awaken, sleep paralysis would set in. I'd plunge into a panic, unable to move. The struggle of trying to lift a finger was so extreme that I would start weeping. My mind was stuck between the dreaming world and the real world. These nightmares haunted me for most of my childhood, and I never told anyone. How could I? I failed to wrap my own head around them.

Trauma keeps you oblivious to why certain things occur in your life. You start to wonder what's wrong with you.

Why don't I fit in?

Why am I treated this way?

Will I ever be normal?

It seems like you're living in a different universe than the people around you. Well, at least that was my experience.

Behind my mask, I was an unsettled child. I'd say I was five years behind my colleagues. Attending more than one elementary school, three different middle schools, and three different high schools further delayed my growth. It was hard for me to mature. How do you catch up to your age when you're forever on the move? As the new girl all the time and never adjusting to the norm, people bullied me. Girls used to schedule to fight me at recess, and I remember hiding behind the bushes in tears of fear. Females hated me, and I didn't know why.

I had trouble making and sustaining real friendships as I aged, and whenever they did accept me into the popular clique, I was pushed to the lowest rank—the one who was the most puppet-like. I did everything to please others, no matter how degrading it looked.

Flaws in my appearance were discovered after joining the cheerleading and dance team. My complexion wasn't as toned as the other girls, my skin wasn't as beautiful, and my chest wasn't as perfect.

My thought processing and conversational skills were inadequate. Bright and brainy when it came to schoolwork, but socially awkward to say the least. Grade school was a low and lonely place for me. I was misread, inferior, and vulnerable. Because of this, my soul yearned for some sort of haven. I needed to tap into a realm where I could let go of my emotions.

Flipping through the channels on television, I came across a lesbian film at eleven years old. The images aroused me. With my eyes plastered to the screen in awe, I masturbated for the first time. The hormones released from my brain gave me an unexplainable high. Peace and relaxation flooded my body like never before, and I drifted off to sleep. From that day forward, it became an addiction of mine. I needed it all the time. With the issues I faced in finding my identity, masturbation allowed me to connect with my body. To find myself again, even if it was just for a second. Nights didn't pass without doing it, and after many sessions, I found a way to be pleased without watching porn. My subconscious persuaded me that I was taking back what was stolen from me as a child. Was I taking it back, though? No. I was just abusing myself all over again.

While the evenings were filled with pleasure, the mornings after were filled with guilt. I thought people were scanning the mystery behind my eyes. That type of shame brought me into my worst isolation. I did whatever I could to blend in because I was afraid of being exposed, including letting people treat me badly and not knowing how to stand up for myself. In some cryptic logic, I believed it to be my punishment for sinning.

Dealing with this obsession behind closed doors changed the hardwiring of my brain. Those of us who are victimized by private sexual sin have no idea what we are doing to ourselves on the inside. The performance is gratifying, so we continue the actions over and over again. Next thing you know, the brain and body have created a dependence: the sex crave that never dies. This crave can lead to physical and mental ruin, and the harm is greater if you begin at a young age when the brain is still growing.

Porn and masturbation can cause at least two effects:

1. You develop a higher risk of contracting depression and anxiety. Endorphins, dopamine, serotonin, and oxytocin are released. The more you engage, the more you give off those chemicals. The more those chemicals are released, the higher the chance of an imbalance.

2. The euphoria that you experience will fashion a "supernormal stimulus"—which is an artificial product that elicits amplified versions of our natural reactions to sex. This creates an unfulfilling sex life because anything less than fantasy won't quench your thirst.

After being raped and bullied and psychologically abusing myself, I loathed who I had become. I wanted to be somebody else, anyone else. I hated being in this strange piece of flesh, and I grew envious of other girls who had it all together, the girls who were lucky enough to be mentally stable. Sin drowned me. I had the outer frame of a kind, Christian girl, yet the inner portions of a demonic spirit. Self-blame attacked my thoughts, and the confusion made me believe I was born to be a homosexual, masturbating addict. Identifying as that woman for years broke me. But opening up about my secrets was not an option. I was afraid of getting into massive trouble or being viewed as a sick person.

What if I'm the only one struggling with this? What if this makes me look crazy?

Not wanting to risk it, I hid it.

Fast forward to 14 years old, the age I had heterosexual intercourse for the first time. He was much older than me, and the typical unfaithful guy. Our breakup unleashed a new low. Childhood boyfriends disrespected me, heightened my self-consciousness, and made me feel like I was competing for their love. I made it easy for them to do whatever they desired because sex kept them coming back for more. It was my superpower. Sex was probably the reason I invited other forms of transgression as well. Smoking, drinking, swearing, and partying became huge chunks of my life, a life that gratified me. Sin was winning. Why would I return to purity?

My story should not come as a shock to you. Molestation mutated the cells in my body, and I became a carcinogenic mess. I'd say a mental breakdown was begging to eat me alive and spit out the bones. I was a helpless, broken crayon. Something that once lit up a room with joy was placed in the hands of a young woman who mishandled it for her pleasure.

ACT
on this!

Sometimes, all roads lead
back to your childhood. What
are some childhood experiences
that could have contributed
to your mental illness?

IF LITTLE OL' DAVID COULD CUT OFF THE HEAD OF HIS GIANT, CERTAINLY I COULD WIN THE FIGHT AGAINST MY OWN.

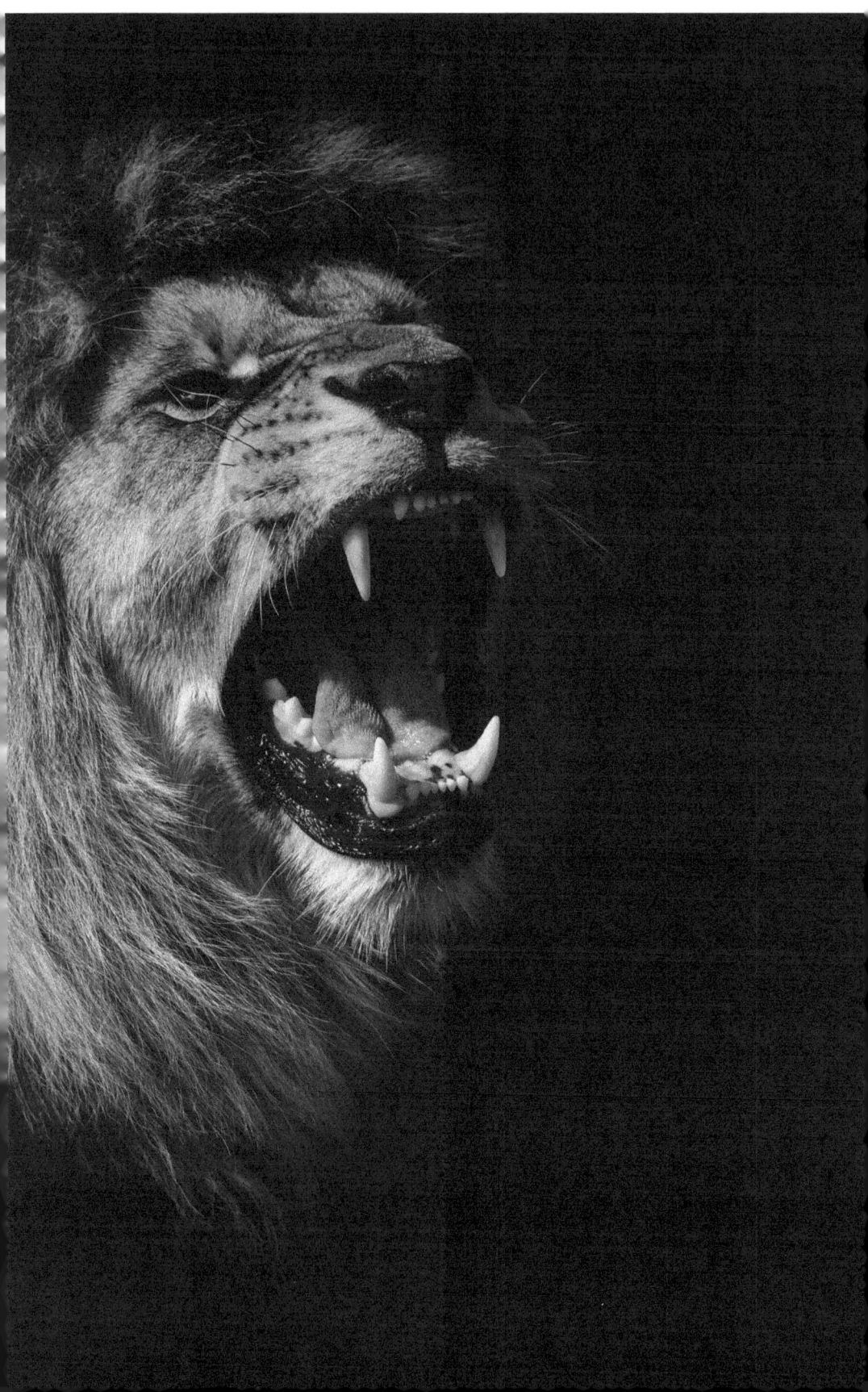

CHAPTER THREE

FACING GOLIATH

My growth produced a lot of demons. But God's grace flourished me. That's the beautiful thing about God. No matter your weakness, He tends to burn right through it. He allowed people to see the external light, not the internal fight. My husband was one of those people. He noticed the glow from the beginning, and he captured it. He took my advice, added points to his character, and leaped forward in life. Unfortunately for me, the more light he obtained, the dimmer I became. My greatness was eclipsed by his. Everyone glorified his jump shots while I sat on the sidelines, waiting for my chance to play.

It was embarrassing to hear myself beg for attention:

"Can you not see me standing here as well?"

Not one person saw me next to him. I was transparent. The dirt underneath his shoes. Day after day, I wished to crop out the unwanted memories and reset to default. We went from being passionately in love to standing on opposite sides of a brick wall. I never saw this coming. The extinguished butterflies, I mean.

We were stapled together at the beginning of our relationship. Wyll was the finest human I had ever laid eyes on. I was crazy in love with that man. He had the perfect smile, the sexy skin tone, the sense of humor, and the compassion to match. I treasured him. We spent mornings, afternoons, and late nights joined at the hip. Everything about our relationship was perfect, the intimacy, the conversations, the mini-dates, the sex. Yes, even the sex was good. We couldn't seem to get enough of it. But too much of a good thing is never *really* good. Is it? Soon enough, we reaped what we had sown. The downfall of our obsession was the tiny humans that made an early debut.

Our first pregnancy was intentional. I remember us being in the heat of the moment when we realized there were no more condoms. We stopped and looked at one another, then made an ignorant decision...

"If it happens, we'll just take care of it."

My naïve teenaged thinking supposed that getting an abortion was an okay thing to do. Society made abortions no different than a yearly pap, so I considered it. The following month, there was a surprise knocking at my door. I spent a lot of time at

Wyll's dorm when he began to spot a few changes in me. I was exhausted. My body felt weird. I couldn't keep anything down.

Lying next to me while watching our favorite show, he said the words no teenager wants to hear, "Baby, I think you're pregnant."

While I tried to ignore the signs, I could not bring myself to disagree with him. I later headed to Walmart to buy a pregnancy test. A positive sign appeared immediately after peeing on the stick. Though I was prepared for this to happen, it stunned me when I saw the results in my hands. I guess it was the nature of a mother that kicked in, knowing that a baby chose to grow in me. I sat there in my feelings for a minute. Then I thought, *I'm only 18 years old. My mom will kill me if I keep this child.*

The fear led to an internet search for abortion clinics and a scheduled appointment after that. Upon arriving at the clinic, something felt off. I was anxious about the process.

I couldn't help but think, *How do they hurt the baby? Could I really die from this? Will I be able to have kids in the future?*

Hesitation set in. I didn't want to go through with it. But I was afraid of how my life would turn out if I didn't. When they invited me back into the exam room to measure the baby, they asked if I wanted to view the ultrasound. I declined the offer. I could not bear to see something that was about to be vacuumed out of me. I felt awful. After the ultrasound, they escorted me to the area where the procedure would take place. There was a plethora of reclining chairs with many young women sitting in them. I got to my chair, and they knocked me out with anesthesia. Although I hated what I had done, I was happy for it to be over.

Life resumed as normal after the school break. Well, if you consider a second pregnancy right after an abortion to be normal. In August of 2011, our method of protecting became the method of breaking. The rubbers that we depended on let us down. You hear the horror stories about condoms ripping on people all the time, but you never believe it could happen to you. I was shattered when I found out it had broken. Our luck failed us. I took another pregnancy test on Wyll's 21st birthday and revealed the news to him over the phone that night. Our conversation ended in my choice to keep our child. Maybe it was God trying to tell me that everything was in His hands. Or perhaps it was just a guilty conscience. Either way, I knew I was keeping this one. Wyll respected my decision and promised to do whatever he could to care for us. Witnessing his maturity was a relief, and it helped me tell my family. A few hours later, we were making the calls.

I trembled as I dialed my mother's number. She flipped. Worry and disappointment caused her to discuss termination. That was a likely response, I guess. After all, I was the first of her children to ever attend college. Not to mention her first daughter. Afraid of telling her about the abortion and refusing to go down that route again, I shut down her advice.

"I can't do that, Mom. I want to keep it."

She explained that she would not be taking care of us if I made that decision. Her voice ascended as she warned me about the difficulties I would face. Anxiety took over my mind, and I ran out of words to say.

My husband stepped in on my behalf. "I'll take care of her and our baby. I'll drop out of school, get a job, and make sure she gets her degree. This is my promise to you."

My mother told each of my siblings after the call. Not even 10 minutes later, they were buzzing in and giving us the same talk. I heard it all and ignored it all. The one thing I was sure of this time around was that I refused to abort this baby. Now, not all of our family's responses were the same. Wyll's mother was our final call.

She cried in excitement when she found out and invited us to stay with her. Four months later, we packed up our dorms, said our goodbyes, and drove four hours north. Wyll began working the night shift in Atlanta while I stayed home. When I was living there, my pregnancy turned into an illness wrapped inside of a uterus. I hated leaving the bedroom, spending time with his family, and doing simple things for myself. I ate and showered. That was all. I had no idea what was happening to me. Inwardly, I felt chaotic. On the outside, I just looked pregnant. My blown-up belly hid the mental deterioration, so it was hard to explain my solitude. The undiagnosed depression was probably a mixture of things: my childhood, my lost identity, the absence of my family, and crazed hormones.

The failure to justify my slump dug a tunnel in our relationship. Deep conversations turned into black arguments. We often questioned the amount of love we had left, but thankfully, not the presence of our love. We wanted this to work, despite our problems. For it to work, we had to commit, to see from each other's perspectives, and to marry. Sealing the knot under God's throne mattered the most to me. Forget the white dress and the flower girl, I wanted to birth our baby under a covenant. Simple and sinless did the job.

We found a one-bedroom apartment in north Georgia a month before our baby arrived. Our move-in date was scheduled for July, so we stayed with my mother until it was ready. She and I strengthened our relationship over the length of my pregnancy, and she wanted to help me post-birth. Although a generous offer, those eight weeks were bumpy. The experience of becoming a first-time mother was nothing like they said it would be. No one ever tells you that postpartum is really post-you. I gave myself away when I had my daughter. My only purpose was to feed my baby, change her, bathe her, and repeat. I hated the bi-hourly feeding that bruised my nipples, the back pain from the epidural, the fictional state of sleep, the restroom sessions that involved me strapping her to my chest, and the times I made a mistake. The uncertainty of motherhood created a film of downcast, and I dreaded the day I would have to go it alone.

Moving into our place did not erase this apprehension. Moving put me in a shock that I never recuperated from. Everything attached to me was new. A new home. A new baby. A new marriage. From 2012 to 2017, I went through what I call "boxed-up" depression and anxiety. Inside of the boxes was hidden evidence of mental illness, but on the outside was the title: Life happens. Life happened so fast for me, faster than I could wrap my head around it. I know what it feels like to be forced into a role before you're mentally prepared for it. I have lived out the expression *age is nothing but a number*. You are as old as you psychologically feel. At twenty, I still felt fifteen. My mind was trapped in the ninth grade while my body was taken into a future I could not handle.

One minute, I was a child still learning how to drive. The next, I was the guardian of a human who entrusted me with her life. My responsibilities frightened me. I wanted to be the very best mother a kid could have and the best wife to my husband. Yet it was all too much. I wasn't primed for the pressure. Instead of being my husband's partner, I became inferior to him. Submission was a term I did not accept right away. It seemed as though my opinions about our life had no effect, as if "I do" erased my independence. Two of the smallest words in the dictionary were two of the most impactful words of my adulthood. I lost myself when I found him. Marriage deleted the goodness of my character, and I was robbed of my twenties. We were the two young people in Hell who were grinding their teeth in anguish while the majority had the option to be selfish. Demons prospered from tormenting us. We lived in a wrestling match, always fighting for peace of mind.

Wyll's job added to our stress. He went from being laid off his night shift job to accepting a position requiring weekly travel and weekend calls. His career placed a burden on our marriage, finances, and personal life. We were a middle-class family who made too much for governmental help, while at the same time living paycheck to paycheck. The promotions were never enough, as our bills swallowed every dollar that hit our account. We were broke. We were distant. The empty pockets created an emptiness between us. Arguing became our native communication, and hatred became our way to love. Sex was even a foreign act in the bed.

My husband was so consumed with providing for me that he neglected his attention toward me. He was absent—physically and emotionally. I barely saw his face, and when he was on the road, we never spoke. A phone call with him was more like a phone call with his job. Screaming at the top of my lungs from the torment of separation anxiety was a *day in the life* for me. There was hardly a time we had an actual conversation without an opening debate.

Unable to spend quality time with my husband for five years worsened my mental health. I was constipated with sweet talks that never happened and moments that were never released. He was either not listening, shutting down, telling me he would speak with me later, or drifting off to sleep. It hurt to be rejected by the one I loved. I sobbed for his attention. Getting excited to see his name show up on my call log or for his presence to appear at the front door resulted in void. It was never really him. It was the overworked, gloomy man that a stupid profession made him out to be. Divorce climbed to the top of my wishlist, as I regretted ever meeting my husband. We became enemies who shared room and board.

That period of my life also welcomed a never-ending tsunami of questioning my purpose. For as long as I can remember, I had dreamed of becoming a top physician in the country. Before taking off in that direction, though, a family member stopped me.

She said to study as a nurse first and then decide later if medical school is still an option. I took the advice, but nursing wasn't a good fit. Whenever I leaped forward in my career, something would pull me down.

At the beginning of my nursing program, my scores were off the charts. They were so high that I was inducted into one of the most prestigious honor societies and given a scholarship. During the last half of the program, my smile had to be drawn on with a blade. The doors of success were slammed shut, multi-locked, and the keys planted six feet under.

My diseases began to manifest in my physical body and caused me dismissal from the program. Twice in under two years, I failed out. Anxiety had trickled down to my fingers during notetaking, making my hands go numb. Depression brought on migraines, fatigue, incoherence, and memory loss. Funding for my education was even cut off. Everything that could go wrong, did. It was over in the blink of an eye. The achievement meter that was once burning up hot fell below the freezing point and shattered in my face. I could feel myself rip in half.

What did I do wrong?

Is it really over?

How am I going to tell my husband that I failed a second time?

I was a disgrace. I couldn't stand to look in the mirror without wanting to commit suicide. The plans I had were a figment of my imagination. Being a mother changed me. Getting married changed me. Getting kicked out of school changed me. None of it was for the better. It was for the worse.

I blamed a major part of my decline on my husband pressuring me to get pregnant a second time. Although I love my baby, Josiah's birth placed a heavier weight on my shoulders. Over the years, I've had trouble raising my daughter. She has a rebellious, fearless attitude that I try to master. Spankings, timeouts, soft explanations, loud yelling, and taking things away prove ineffective. With prophetic gifting on her life, I learned that she would always be more of a handful than your typical American child. But knowing this never fixes it. Raising a prophet doesn't come with a blueprint. After countless botched attempts, our relationship began to sink when she was ending her toddler years. I couldn't stand to be around her. I wanted to avoid the backtalk, smirks, and disobedience. Of course, no one understood this.

People confused my frustration for lack of love and patience toward my daughter. That was far from the truth. I was exhausted, weary of belittlement by a child I chose to birth, one whose life I fought for. Any like-minded mother in my shoes would have felt defeated. When she was about three years old, I decided that she would be an only child. My husband disagreed. He thought a sibling would help to stabilize her. I rejected the idea, he called me selfish for not wanting more, and I surrendered to his will in the end. Why? Because I was afraid of him cheating on me and getting another woman pregnant.

Following my son's birth, Kaelyn grew worse, and so did I. Forty pounds heavier than my pre-pregnancy weight, loosened abs that never went back to normal, and stretch marks to seal the deal.

I was done. For a woman who has tussled with body dysmorphia their whole life, this was enough to make me explode. I broke the record of my depression from 2017 to the end of 2018. That's when I finally diagnosed myself as being mentally ill.

After leaving college, someone placed a thousand books on the stop button of life. Going on an intense journey to find the best job for my family left me applying for every position that matched my history. Doing this was a total drain of energy, though. Not one company called or emailed me to schedule an interview. I wasn't even qualified for waitressing and working at the mall, apparently. My husband and I believed it might have been a sign that I needed to be available for our kids and work from home, so I pursued every at-home job and career out there—from personal assisting to modeling. Modeling was the one pursuit that seemed promising, but it did more harm than good to my character. The criticism made me obsess over my appearance. I scoured the pages of influencers on Instagram and fell in love with the beautiful structure of their faces, *Maybe if my nose was this small, people would love me. If my cheekbones were like hers, I could gain respect.*

Their likes, comments, and followers were the circus tickets for the world of attraction, but my stats granted me popcorn on the couch as I viewed from a distance, wishing I could look like them. I hated myself and no longer saw the reason I existed. The floor cracked underneath me and inhaled my body through its nostrils. All that remained was the unfertilized egg waiting in my mother's uterus for someone to give me a chance at life. As the ovum, I unplugged. Depression electrocuted me until my nerves ripped apart. He blinded me from reality by gauging my eyes out. He sewed my mouth shut to counteract my power to expose him. He unzipped my spine and left me as mush.

My life consisted of swimming in oceans of tears and desiring to harm myself. I was hesitant if I would make it through the day without having a mental breakdown. I fought the urge to kill myself, afraid to keep on living, but more afraid of death. With a trillion negative thoughts playing on repeat in my head, insomnia won me over at night. I longed to die in my sleep. Getting out of bed in the mornings hurt. I dreaded to live another day in isolation and disappointment. But if I remained in bed, my kids would not get fed. So, I walked lazily to the bathroom each morning, trying to gain the stamina to get ready for the day. The toilet was my throne of thought. I could sit there until my legs became strangled by the absence of circulation. It was my center for processing what was happening. Tears would moisten my palms as I rooted my face in my hands. After gathering myself together, I would enter the shower. The shower was my favorite part of the day because it cried with me. In those borders, I felt secure. After sobbing under the stream of water until my throat began to hurt, I'd exit the door and head to my final destination, the mirror of truth.

This massive piece of glass provided a clear reflection of an unclear direction. It showed my insignificance. I vividly saw the words: failure, ugly, fat, a nobody, and unloved written across my forehead in black sharpie. I searched for every flaw in my face and tried to contour my nose skinnier, my cheeks slimmer, my eyes more defined, and my lips more prominent. I wanted to cover up the words on my forehead with a full-coverage concealer. I hid my depressed scars with the swipe of a brush. Mental illness abused me. Its hands crucified me.

My clock went in reverse until I became a baby again, learning to crawl. I underperformed at everything my fingers touched. I lost memory of the most basic concepts, even forgetting my home address. The cloudiness of my thoughts made me drop the lightest object out of my hands, as small as a toddler toothbrush. I became weak. I was psychologically and physically anemic. With my weakness came self-harm. I punished myself by not eating some days. I scratched my legs until sores appeared whenever I had a breakdown. I drove carelessly, hoping that I would run off the road and make it look like an accident. This illness had it out for me, and in return, I had it out for myself. I dreaded being in this capsule. I was tired of being powerless. How much more could a person take? I figure depression was wondering the same thing because I continued to suffer. He wanted to see how long I'd last before I caved in to death.

As I metaphorically sat in the back of an unmarked van blindfolded and tied up by depression, I heard a second voice. The voice of anxiety. He entered me and fed off of me like a virus. You see, a virus can only gain its power from a living organism. It cannot do much by itself. For a virus to infect anything, a host is needed, and they'll do whatever they can to find one. The instant they take control over your cells, the door is opened for more to enter your body. The same is true for conditions in the brain.

Imagine that there's a room full of mental disorders with a door that keeps them locked in. They're waiting to be released, but they need to find a living organism. You are the wanted candidate. You happen to be walking past the room, heading to your next destination when they feel the heatwave of your presence slide underneath the door. The aroma of your innocence turns them on, and they break into a brawl over who will get to take you home. They're like men lusting after a woman. The second that door opens, one of them begins to prey on you. At that point, you are no longer your own. You are their property.

It was depression who date-raped me first. He worked to limit me until my strength was wrecked. Because I became so frail, anxiety saw me as a target. Anxiety was the copycat killer who partnered with depression to skin me alive. He made my heart race from China to Mars in 0.01 seconds. He forced me to avoid social gatherings, and if I disobeyed, he would cause tremors in my hands, shakiness in my voice, memory loss, and a hole in my throat. He instilled random thoughts of terror in my head of cars crashing into me or someone shooting me from behind. Every so often, I would get beatings by him. He would attack my breathing, remove the oxygen from my body, and cause migraines to leave me vomiting into the toilet. He also tortured me by whispering negativity about my past, making me scrutinize any situation that left me feeling self-conscious. Both depression and anxiety were my slaveowners. I wasted many lonely days and nights sitting in a daze for hours at a time because I could no longer feel. The aches numbed me. I tried reaching out for my husband's guidance, but he accused me of being melodramatic. I tried reaching out to my family for help, but they taped a pretty picture over my ugly condition. Someone close to me even went as far as to call me out of my race, as if mental infirmity was color-specific. Falling to my knees was hopeless because I lost my faith. No one had my back, and I wanted to leave the earth.

Then one day, something occurred to me. I realized that all this time, beginning in my childhood, I had come face to face with a giant. I was facing a Goliath. Oddly enough, this reassured me. It reminded me of the famous story from the Bible. Then I thought, *If little ol' David could cut off the head of his giant, certainly I could win the fight against my own.*

The life in this casing of mine was spent. I wanted to take a leap of faith. Doing this on my own was unreasonable, though. I needed help. Serious help. The supernatural help I once believed in.

ACT
on this!

We often don't realize we're fighting a giant until it nearly crushes us. At what point did you notice depression had become your Goliath?

"

I AM NO LONGER MAD AT
GOD FOR ALLOWING ME TO
GO THROUGH PAIN. I AM
THANKFUL, FOR IT WAS
IN THE PAIN THAT I
FOUND PURPOSE.

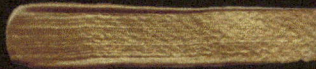

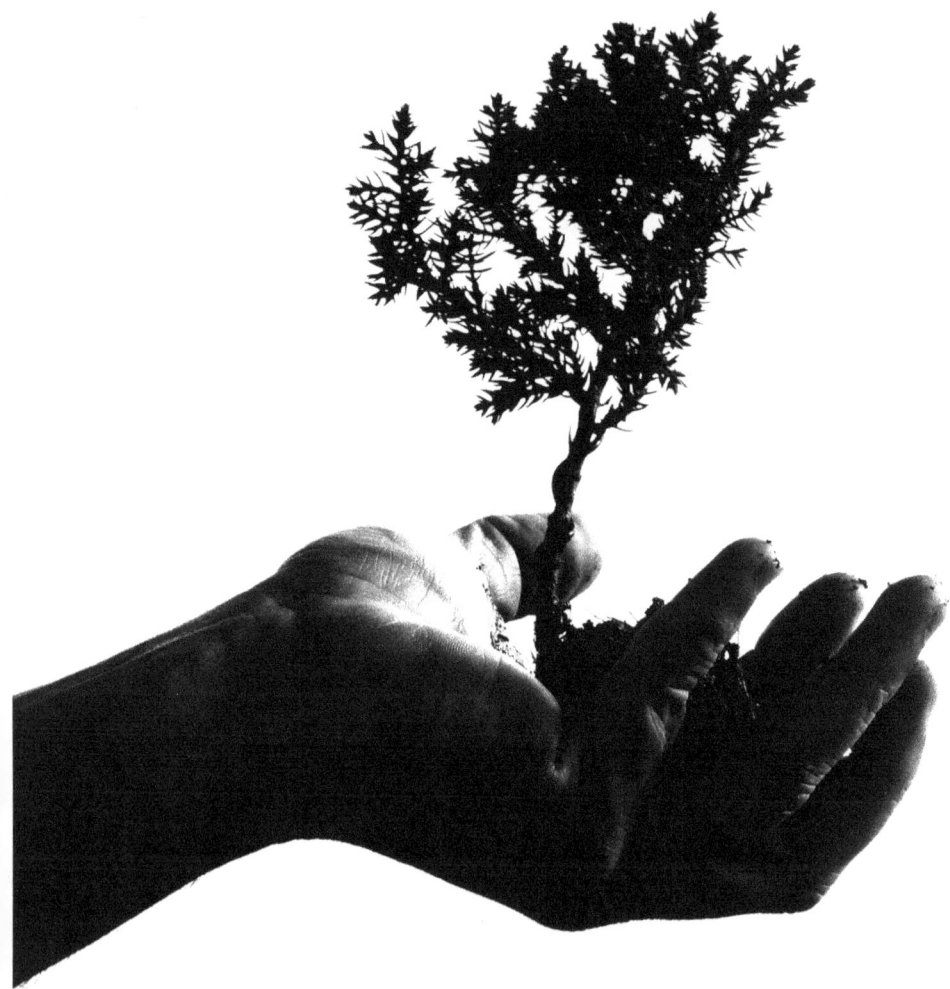

CHAPTER FOUR

THE UNEARTHING

To unearth means to dig deep into the ground and remove something from its root, to discover that which was lost and kept in a secret place. To fish for it, scoop it out, bring it to the surface, reveal it, expose it. When you unearth, you are delivering one of Earth's babies. You're pulling something out of the land and washing off the waxy, cheese-like substance that coated its flesh.

I am very familiar with the process of unearthing. I was once the baby who was drowning in the gunk of an earthly sac. The Lord cast His net wide and found me trying to punch my way through a grave like the scene from *Kill Bill*. He washed me clean, uncovered my identity, and recovered me in His glory. I was born on three different occasions in my lifetime. My natural birth, my freedom birth, and my birth as the Word of God. The first birth was in 1992. The final two happened 27 years later. God delivered me from one realm and into another. For this to make better sense to you, I'll have to walk you through it.

My illness thrust me into the ground. As I laid there with dirt in my lungs and choking on nature, the Spirit of Life showed up. I saw majestic feet standing next to me and tears of pain hitting the ground when a hand reached down and pulled me out. Though it was disguised as a church invite from my apostle, the Lord asked if there was still room for Him.

I will admit, this was not my apostle's first time inviting us back to church. He had done so off and on for a few years, and I rarely showed my face. The truth is, I wanted to be in the presence of God, but I was dodging the emotional ride that it welcomed. Whenever we attended church, my husband received praise and prophecies about job promotions while I was told that God was just visiting my womb. This made me believe my only purposes were to have children and support Wyll's career.

The career that broke us apart.

The career that almost killed me.

Through all of the trials of my identity, my marriage sinking, the parental hardship, and depression, going to church never helped. Avoiding it altogether seemed to be the answer. My mind was made up, and I was set in my ways. But if you know anything about God, you know that His plans for you are always different than your own. He knew what I needed, and the only thing He needed in return was for me to enter His gates. He was going to do the rest.

On December 15, 2018, I decided to bite the bullet and go to church. I had no expectations that I would benefit from the sermon, for I was sure I would leave upset. I walked in and sat on a pew without a thrill. Then out of nowhere, something amazing happened. Instead of me leaving upset, I was set up for the first sign of victory. A guest speaker whom I had never met was ministering to the congregation. The Father must have been waiting on us because not only was the message directed toward me, but he had a personal word to give my family. That day marked the first of 12 prophecies that turned my life downside, up.

The prophet's description of our life was proof that God was in that place. He spoke about the Lord prospering my hands, healing my marriage, increasing our finances, and healing our hearts. I felt my illness take a step backward as I received the word. Tears dropped, and I fell out in the Spirit. I went home rejoicing and thanking God for the work that He was getting ready to do. For about two weeks, I was mentally stable, longer than I had ever been since my depression started. I thought I'd never go back into that darkness again,

"Was that it?" I asked myself. "All I needed to do was go to church?"

Sadly, that wasn't it. I had a greater level to pass. Depression met joy, and they fought over who would get to buy my thoughts. A full auction took place, and depression bought it back for 200, Alex.

How is God going to prosper my hands?

This question loomed until I fell into the trap of thinking I wasn't worthy enough to be blessed. After returning home from dinner one night, a conversation with my husband turned on self-doubt.

I started to blurt out my concerns, "I'll never be good enough. I can't even talk to people without forgetting my words. I can't look in the mirror and feel confident in my own skin. I can't be a good mother to my children, and I can't be good for you. How could I ever be used by God?"

Voices raised and separation commenced. I crawled into an anxiety attack and could not catch my breath. I dug my nails deep into my thighs. Then I ran into the bathroom and cried out, "God, who am I?"

As doubt climbed and fear took control of my body, the Lord answered my call. His voice was mesmerizing:

"Find out everything you can about Me. And in that, I will show you who you are and what your purpose is on this earth."

Although I called out to Him, I wasn't planning on hearing a response. I thought prayer was a one-way conversation. You speak to God and then go about your day, hoping something would change. So, the moment He spoke, I was surprised and relieved. I raised my chin, wiped my face, and departed the bathroom with a newfound strength. I walked into the kitchen and tidied up some last-minute dishes. Jesus walked in behind me. He started cleaning me out as I cleaned out the dishes. I find it funny that the Lord used the environment I cook in to prepare me as a new recipe in Christ.

His presence weakened every part of my body. Chills ran through me, causing the bowl in my hands to fall into the sink, and I wept in His arms. It was like He looked down at me and told me everything was going to be just fine. It was His turn to take over.

The true power of God rested on me that night. Depression and anxiety were ants compared to His pinky finger. With His whole hand? He was getting ready to blow my mind. He delivered me and purposed me all in one night. I felt more alive than ever before. I advanced from three breadths of burden to 18 breadths of protection. The Trinity covered all six sides of me: the front, the back, the left, the right, the top, and the bottom. Multiply a three-dimensional Being by the six borders of a person, and it equals out to be 18 dimensions of security. This is so powerful when you consider 18 to be the numerical value for the Hebrew word *chai*, a word that means "life" in the English language.[1] He was giving life back to me! But it wasn't going to be like before. This life would be off the charts. This life would be a dream made into a reality.

Per the Lord's instruction, I laid out a path to get to know Him. I told my husband what I experienced, and we talked about God's love for the rest of the night. I later went on a quest to purchase a new Bible. The old ones I had were not structured for Bible study. This was a new phase in my life. I needed to walk different. I needed to study deeper. Upon opening the Word, a profound statement in the preface caught my attention. The writer showed me that the Bible is an important piece of gold that defines our identity. She also defended the Creator, saying that He is not responsible for the injustices we meet in this world.[2] The Enemy used a woman to birth sin, but Father counteracted his plan by using another woman to give birth to the Savior.

This agreed with what God told me in the bathroom. I had not known that my identity was based upon the God in me. I supposed we were identified by our physical names, careers, and personality. Reading this confirmed that I did hear His voice that night! The latter portion of the statement was also warming. I misjudged Him in the middle of my downfall. I was sure that He had turned His back on me. Boy, was I wrong. The Lord never orchestrated my illness. Satan did. Now, why would my Father allow him to torture me? Because in order to build me up to the highest place, I had to feel the pain of rejection. Depression gave me endurance. Sadness gifted me everlasting happiness. Anxiety taught me the true meaning of peace.

I pressed forward in the Word. Each verse reminded me that I am who He says I am. His revelation sank into my spirit, and the request for wisdom came to pass. I began to evolve into the scriptures *as* the Scripture. I appreciated God for the quick work that He was doing on the inside. My low thoughts were replaced with bliss. My reckless memory was traded for His knowledge. Self-hatred was substituted for His love. Inability was replaced with His capability. Weakness was traded for His strength. Darkness was replaced with light.

Reading the Word of God started to adjust the chemicals in my brain. I became more like God and less like depression. My spirit was being renewed day after day. My might grew stronger and more resilient. My faith took me back to when I was two years old and believed in His promises. The Father was unearthing me! He pulled out the roots of mental affliction and laid a new groundwork, new soil.

This was it! No more fighting myself. No more fighting my calling. I was forming into a jewel of love. I saw everything differently: my family, myself, God. I loved life! A new me was springing forth, and I was excited to watch her grow.

Near the end of January, I reached out to my apostle. He learned about my struggle recently, and I wanted him to know I was improving. In our next service, He had a word to give me. Prosperity was mentioned again, as well as gaining a strong identity as a mother, wife, and a force for the Kingdom. He also declared that lowliness would never overtake me, and God would provide an explosion of favor. I played that recording numerous times. I also designed a transcription of it, had it framed, and read it aloud until I committed it to memory. I was living out the words of the Bible without knowing it. 1 Timothy 1:18 tells us to recall our prophecies, so we may win the war against our soul. I defeated the horrible words spoken against me using the good word spoken for me. My solid faith produced a hasty turnaround.

A month after that prophecy, I was baptized in the Holy Spirit. Two days later, I received my tongues. A few weeks after that, my spiritual gifts began developing. All of it was sudden. A fast life brought me into sickness. Yet the Lord worked a thousand times faster to reverse it. He was taking me higher than I could have ever gone. He was shaving off my old snakeskin and repairing the atoms in my body to look like His. I changed seasons—from the coldest winter to the happiest summer. God brought me out of one extreme into the next. I went from not being able to speak, to acquiring a life language; unable to see past death, to looking at the mind of God. He balanced out the chemicals in my brain and allowed them to function at a superior level. He had done a new thing in me.

In March, I received a call from my apostle regarding two projects he wanted me to launch. The first was a position in the church. He would have me writing and designing bi-weekly newsletters. The second was this book, an idea that was originally brought to my attention by my husband. After hearing this advice a second time, I knew it was God's plan for me to start writing. Our talk inspired me, and I committed to both projects right away. The newsletters were done quickly, but the book was tiresome. My fear constructed a temporary funeral, and I put the book down. The following weekend, I received another word from the Lord. He gave me the confirmation I needed to finish the manuscript.

When I began writing again, I went through a range of emotions. Finally getting the chance to talk about what I had been through was freeing. But having to relive that cruelty was unfavorable. Many times I doubted my ability to get it done. But the Spirit was my comfort. God has been faithful in keeping His word. He's both empowered me and graced me for each of my callings. No matter how much I hesitated to open up about my private issues, He never failed to remind me of the testimonies in the Bible.

Every vessel used by the Father has an ugly part in their story. That's what makes it a beautiful ending. We are each born into sin. No one person is greater than another. We all fall short. We all need His forgiveness and healing. If the stories in the Bible were crowded with perfection, we would be in trouble. There'd be no evidence of God performing the impossible. There would be no reason for Him to do a new thing. His qualifications would plainly state:

Undetermined, experience pending, skills unknown.

If a testimony leaves out the presence of a test, what good is it for people who need inspiration? How would we know He's a Healer, if He's never had the opportunity to heal a woman from cancer? How would we know He's a Deliverer, if He's never had the chance to free a man from addiction? How would we know He's a Savior, if there was no one left to save? Testimonies have to be told. It is the raw story of God's children that encourages others to believe—to keep the faith, to fight. The Bible is full of product reviews that conclude, "If God did it for me, He'll do it for you, too!"

David killed and cheated. God used him as a brilliant psalmist. Paul was a persecutor of the Gospel. God used him to author nearly half of the New Testament. Peter denied our Savior. God used him to spread the Gospel. They were sinners who were made alive by the Spirit. Because of their test, we have proof that God comes through, and He prepares us for a life that glorifies Him.

The Father, being One of perfect truth, life, love, wisdom, sufficiency, kindness, justice, grace, mercy, holiness, glory, and beauty, surely has the power to conquer our greatest battle.

God plus nothing still equals everything. God plus depression equals progression. I was a lost soul who was raped, addicted to masturbation, and strangled by Satan, but Jesus has found great use for me. And if He did it for all of us, will He not do it for you? He's been there all along. Though I could not see it, He had plans to mend my marriage, raise my children, free me, and give me a name. I am no longer angry at God for allowing me to go through pain. I am thankful, for it was in the pain that I found purpose. There is nothing more that I could want. I have it all in knowing Him.

As the name "Satan" connected to our mental illness, the name of the Lord challenges it:

Locked

On

Regenerated

Deliverance

Our servanthood to Him guarantees us to be locked on regenerated deliverance. His authority to deliver us out of trouble is loaded on 100 percent every time we call on Him. A fresh batch of grace is made new in Heaven any time you get sick. The Lord is the Operator. His angels are the first responders. His hand is the defibrillator. His glory is the oxygen tank. His blood is the transfusion. His body is the organ donation. He wears every hat according to your degree of need. He's the neurosurgeon, the psychiatrist, the therapist, and the pharmacist. When you reach out to Him, know that you're reaching out to a full range of specialists. He has felt it all. He has healed it all. No mountain of yours is too great. No concern of yours is too small. Trust what I am telling you today. I am a walking testimony of His goodness.

I went from wanting to commit suicide to writing a book about my deliverance four months later. I did not step foot in a counselor's office or take any medication. The Lord cured me. He grabbed me and hugged me so tight that His blood ran through my veins and healed my soul.

ACT
on this!

In Isaiah 43:19, God says, "Behold, I will do a new thing, and it shall spring forth." What new things are you looking for Him to do concerning you? After you've written down your answer, give it to Heaven. Then write the following message on top of yours in big, bold letters: "I AM GOING TO DO SO MUCH MORE THAN THAT." -GOD

"

YOU WERE

PERFECT BEFORE

THE SUBSTITUTIONS.

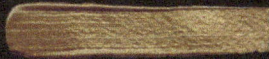

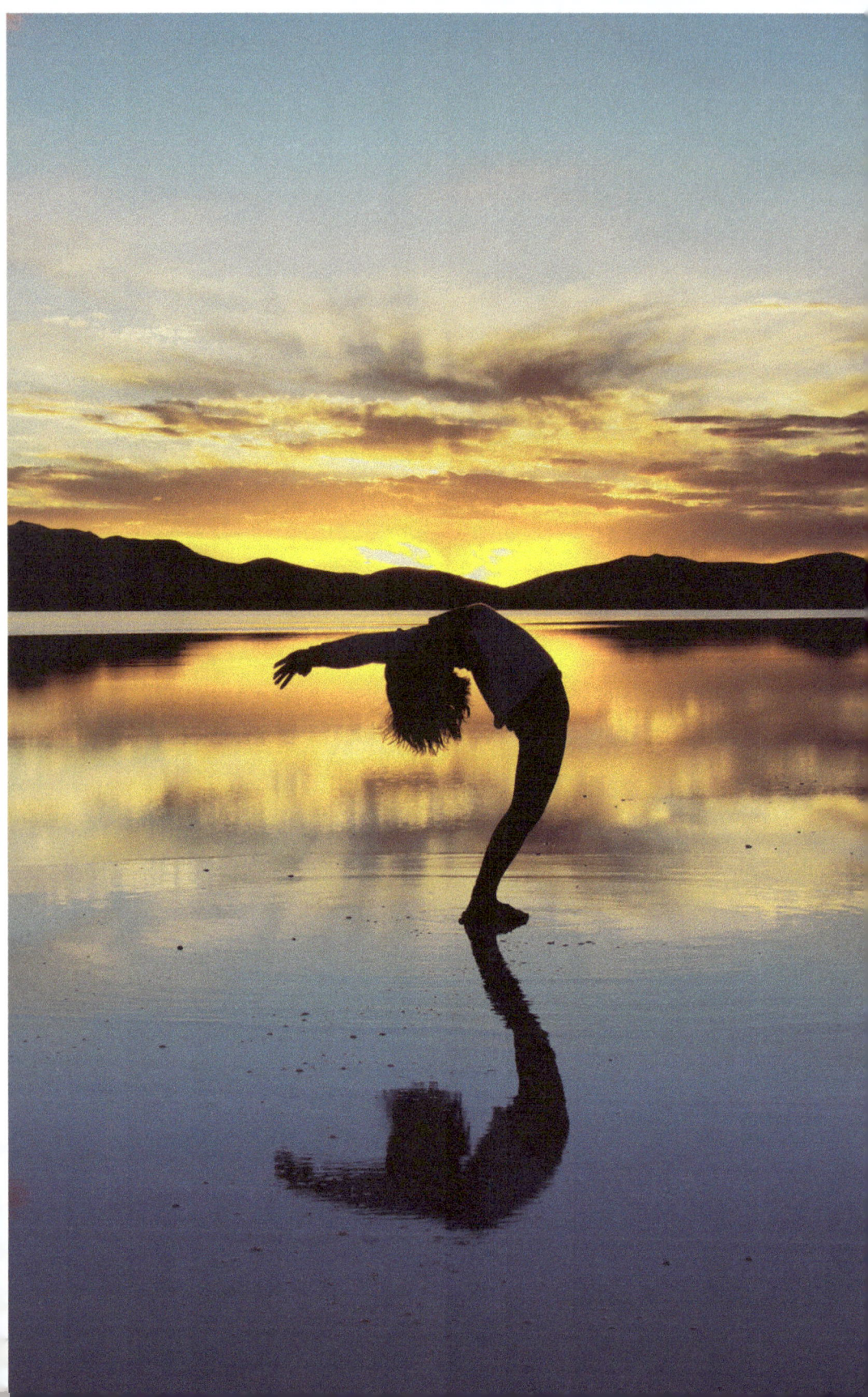

CHAPTER FIVE

THE CONCEPTION PHASE

In the Beginning

n the beginning, God created you, all that you see of yourself and all that you do not see. As time passed, you began to feel like a soup of nothingness—a bottomless pit. The Spirit is brooding over you like a bird above the watery abyss. God is setting you apart from darkness and activating light. He is producing a work of greenery in your life. You will harvest fruit-bearing trees of many kinds. Rivers will flood your belly. He will bless you to prosper, reproduce, and influence. He will look at what He has made and be proud of the woman you have become. The Enemy spoke death. God speaks life.

He says, "I've taken a good look at your afflictions. I've heard your cries for deliverance, and I know all about your pain. I've come to deliver you out of trouble. I've come to shift you from living in the minimum to reaching your maximum potential in Me. I am going to use you to do a mighty work. And when you lack the confidence and wonder why I chose you, remember that I AM with you. I've made every part of the human body, which means I have control over it. That brain of yours? Yes, I can fix that. That low self-esteem? I can change that. That confusion of identity? Give it to me. I'll take care of it. I am the Lord your God. I will instruct your every move. So get up, and let's go! Live your life to the fullest. Give it your heart and soul. And don't for one minute forget what I've promised you. Ponder and meditate on My breath day and night, making sure to put the Word in action. Be strong and courageous, daughter. Don't be timid or downhearted. I am with you every step of the way." (Inspired by Genesis, Exodus, and Joshua)

The Father gave me this prophetic revelation in Bible study one day. I was in the middle of reading John when the Holy Ghost led me to the books of Genesis, Exodus, and Joshua. He said to take you back to the beginning where it all started, to show that you've been activated into the Word, as the Word. Although Genesis is written about earth, it is very well written about you: "As it is in heaven, so it is on earth." (see Matthew 6:10) Better yet, as it is in Heaven, let it be done in you. You are the earth He is speaking of. You were present in the beginning—once covered in darkness; once emptied. But when He arrived as the Light of life, you became the Light as well. Father hoped you would remember home.

Then, a disorder stole your birthright. He could no longer recognize you, so He made a plan, "I have to save her. And the best way to do that is to reform her."

Think of it like this: You are a pot of stew. God is the Chef who made you. Before your conception, He put together a recipe that included the right amount of seasoning. He tasted you and saw that you were good. Then you were placed on the menu for all to witness. Depression ordered you and began to request substitutions: a little less salt, a little more spice. You later became something the Chef could not identify. You became something that lost its original flavor. But God is reminding you today that you were perfect before the substitutions. You were made whole. You are invaluable. He's come down to claim you as His own again. He's come to disclose your entitlement to the largest Kingdom that ever lived, the Kingdom of Heaven.

Before I dive into this concept, let's lay some ground rules first. If by any chance you don't believe in God, I'd like to shed some light on the matter, because rebirth is a whole lot easier when you trust in the Maker.

The subject of God is forever questioned. People want to know how He formed, how long He's been around, and whether or not He truly is the Creator of the universe. Allow me to break off that incertitude. A few months ago, I watched an episode of the *700 Club* that broadened my faith and my opinion of science as a whole. An astrophysicist named Hugh Ross wrote a book explaining how science can prove the existence of God. He was raised as a nonbeliever and spent his childhood learning physics and researching the character of stars. At 16, He aligned with the Big Bang theory, "If the universe was created out of a big bang, then it must have had a beginning. If it had a beginning, then it must have had a Beginner."[1]

That idea motivated Ross to search for the possibility of a God. He read many books on religion, looking for answers, but the Bible was the only Book that had the simplest key to the formation of life. There *was* a Force outside of the walls of the universe that created it all, including time and space.

Ross wanted more. He wanted to seek physical answers and compare them with the spiritual. How in the world would that be possible? The genius of technology. He used imaging devices that allowed him to watch the universe form 13.8 billion years ago. He witnessed nature and Genesis being paralleled to the six-day time frame that God performed His most excellent work. The record of Scripture and science aligned to the tee.

After finishing the experiment, Ross realized another major solution. There would not be a planet earth if the universe wasn't its exact size. Nor if the planet wasn't in its rightful location. Approximately 50 billion, trillion stars make up a quarter of a percent of the cosmos. If there was an extra half of a star or a reduced number of stars by a decimal point, life would be unknown. If Earth was just a fraction closer to the sun, we would all burn. Any further away? We would freeze to death.

The precision of everything, the planets, the stars, the people, the creatures above, below, and on the land, was in the divinity! Not in nature's ability. One Being served as the answer to it all. That perfection conceived us and filled us with the first act of grace. 2 Timothy says, "Grace was given [to] us in Christ Jesus *before* the beginning of time…" This means the Father planned to save us and call us before He made a single thing to do so. That Plan became the Scientific Method for the world accepted. Hear this truth and be set free today:

God…is…real.

Now that we have illustrated the Father of Genesis, let us reveal our link to His genealogy. First off, meet Christ. My main Man. The Universal Ingredient. All things were made through Him, and without Him, nothing was made. He was in the marrow of the Father before He came to us. They were merged as One. John reveals this at the start of his book, "In the beginning was the Word, and the Word was with God, and the Word was God." "…the Word [then] became flesh and dwelt among us…" Jesus's inborn name is the Word of God, for Revelation says, "He is clothed in a robe dipped in blood, and His name is called The Word of God." That is to say, the Father and the Son have the same DNA. Never mind the two separate names. We, too, share the same glory seed, in such a way, that He loved us enough to wear our sufferings. When the Messiah walked the planet, He was the Word of God transformed into our pain, the kind of pain that has defined your past, the kind of pain that you're hurting from right now. Christ downgraded Himself for a short time to upgrade us for a lifetime. He became you to rename you. He worked to replenish you as His own flesh and blood, to apply a full system reboot on your behalf, to redesign you from scratch. If there is one thing He knows how to do extremely well, it is to make something out of nothing.

I was sore when depression left me as scraps, but it felt amazing when the Lord singlehandedly collected those particles and rebirthed me as a shiny new human. He picked me up and said, "That's enough of that. It's time for a reawakening."

He then called me by a name I'd never heard before. He named me the Activated Word. The moment that chorus left His lips, a pregnancy occurred on the inside. I survived three phases of preparation before my activation like a mother endures three trimesters before holding her new creation.

Three. That's all it took. If you ask me, I'd say that's no coincidence—given the symbolism behind that number in Scripture. *Completion* and *unity* are the original meanings of three. The first model of this is the Trinity, but further evidence can be traced. The New Testament, in which rebirth is a major theme, is composed of 27 books. The number 27 is the sum of multiplying three times itself, three different times (3x3x3). The New Testament involves the completion of a person to the third power, making rebirth a tri-completion suite. We also find ourselves breathing in the box of three. The Lord sealed us with a spirit, a soul, and a body and saw us as the finished product. There was such a joy in the completion of man that He went as far as to promote that product on the cross in the format of three.

It is finished were the triad of words that gave fire to that which was dead, and a path to that which was lost. Not to mention, He prayed for three hours in the garden to gain the strength needed to say those words during His torture. As I said prior, God does everything in precision, even in the reports of His physical death.

He was believed to be placed on the cross at the third hour of the day, or 9 a.m., and He died at three in the afternoon (the ninth hour of the day). God is also the only Being who can exist in three tenses of grammar at once: "…peace from Him Who is, and Who was, and Who is to come." (Revelation 1:4) On a further note, He is the only One capable of monopolizing the three characteristics of all-ness: an omniscient God, or all-knowing; an omnipotent God, or all-powerful; and an omnipresent God, manifesting everywhere at all times.

Additional references of three include: Peter's denial of Christ three times, the resurrection on the third day, the fathers of the Israelite nation (Abraham, Isaac, and Jacob), the three scopes of Heaven (Paul visits the third Heaven), and lastly, only three angels are mentioned in the Bible (Lucifer, Michael, and Gabriel).

As you can see, three carries an order, impact, and weight like no other—chiefly in the timetable of humans. The history of humanity is a beacon for the triangle of hope. First a creation, then a fall, then a remake. You are trapped in the fall season of the second stage. Therefore, a rebirth is owed to you in the last. You'll undergo three trimesters before delivery while becoming the Trinity before your deliverance. Let's call it completion to the third power,

3 trimesters before *delivery* = Trinity before *deliverance* = Completion^3

Take a look at our first phase, conception. This word can

be broken down into the prefix *con-* and the suffix *-ception*. Con means with or thoroughly.[2] Ception indicates a nesting, a layering, a recursion.[3] When the two are brought together as one, they come to define conception as thoroughly nesting. The first week of pregnancy is a great example of this. Leading up to implantation, the male's sperm travels along the journey to reach the egg. After one penetrates the ovum, it nests on the inside. The fertilized egg is later taken off the map of possibilities. Meanwhile, the genetic codes from the parents will determine the child's character at once. They are destined to mature into the seed of their family before they even look like them.

Conception is no different with the Word of God. Remember when I said Christ was the Universal Ingredient? I wasn't speaking figuratively. I was speaking literally. Eve wasn't the first to get pregnant. The universe was. Father implanted His Sperm into its ovum, and the Seed had more than enough leverage to split indefinitely, birthing an endless multiplication of life. This is why God sent Jesus to vaccinate us after the crushing. The ground needed a familiar blood to settle in its pores. Earth needed to remember the Program that installed it. Otherwise, it would have rejected every shot to update the prehistoric law. Any old matrix wouldn't have sufficed, and in turn, we would have been eating fire for breakfast, lunch, and dinner. The Word of God substantiated as the Universal Blood Donor. When it tasted Him, the glitches were released, and the unit reset. He handled all the kinks. He printed a new codebook. That same code will overwrite your mental abuse.

When the Word enters your egg, He begins first by piercing your shell, thoroughly nesting in your gut, providing His genetic profile, and placing you on *Satan, do not disturb*. No matter the sum of called-in threats, not one of them will stand against the power of the block. The chemicals of glory will rain on depression's parade. The cavities of death will be subject to life. Your strength will arise. Brightness will become your image. Significance will become your vision.

Supernatural Seed feels like putting on a brand new pair of high heels, a gorgeous set of Christian Louboutins with the red bottoms. Though one of the most expensive brands on the market, it's the color that makes these shoes iconic. Many women purchase them for the status alone. They figure if people can see the red accent, it'll somehow add to their worth. But what's worth more than fitting in a pair of shoes with a real flushed bottom? The brand of Christ. That's what you call attractive. That's a bold and brave female walking, a woman who beats the odds in the red bottoms that have been to Hell and back. She morphs into the strength of her Father by following in His footsteps. Playing dress-up becomes her reality. She takes on His name.

Isn't that what children do anyway? They apply the mask of their parents and carry out the family's name? I still remember when my little girl was two years old. She went through a phase of trying on our shoes. We would laugh hysterically at how adorable she looked in them. It was beautiful to watch her admire us for who we were. We were idols in her eyes. Not too long ago, I came across a picture of her at that age. She had a cute yellow romper on, her hair in two buns with a hat covering them, and her legs hidden inside of her daddy's work boots. She had a ball playing make-believe, though I consider it meant more to her than just cracking a smile on our faces. To my daughter, make-believe was more like make-it-real. Make it last. My baby had a mission, a mission to develop into her parents, the people she viewed as superheroes. You could see the flame in her eyes, determined to honor us by becoming us. She wanted to endorse our names by walking in our shoes. It wasn't the material that mattered the most. It was the words who fit into it. "Mommy and Daddy" was the word duo that she learned first and subscribed to. Those were the words that influenced her character. Whatever we did, she did. Whatever we said, she said. And above all, whatever we called her, she saw herself as.

How powerful is that? The influence of a single word. Your entire life is structured around the words you believe. The world spins on words. Without them, nothing would function. Nothing would exist. Why do you think everything is word-activated? Why do you think you are word-activated? Because if something has a label, it has a solution. God said, "Let there be," and there was. If there are no labels, purpose does not exist.

Light fulfills illumination. The sky establishes hours, days, and seasons. Plants produce seed. Animals contribute to the ecosystem. And if HU is an ancient name for God, as humans, we are God as man.[4] We're the walking breath of God! Everything and everyone is tagged with an assignment. A word is not just an utterance spoken from the mouth. A word is an activated design within itself. Christ takes the prize as the original Word, but you are brushed with those same colors. You match His essence. You fit the shoes that He's made for you, the kind that never breaks, never burdens you, never fades.

So far, we have discussed the first meaning of the word -ception. That mission is launched the moment He nests in your core. The following term related to that suffix is called a layering. This is when God marks you as His own. You become sealed with the Holy Spirit of promise. That seal is like an 850 credit score. No one can deny you. You've earned the right to it all. This makes you fully eligible to receive the three-edged sword that paces with the Spirit—an inheritance of power, love, and a sound mind. The latter cuts mental illness at the neck and burns it until every little ash disintegrates. The first demolishes walls and breaks open the doors that are undefeated by man alone, yet conquerable with the Cornerstone. Love? Well, love is the circuit breaker. Love is the reason this system works. He coated us in grace, He clothed us in royalty, and we beheld His glory, all because of His love.

Isn't it a tender feeling when God asks you to run back into His arms so He can prove this love? I'd run a million miles to receive something so pure. And if I grow weary in the race toward grace, fainting would be illogical. He would meet me in my weakness and offer to carry me the rest of the way. My God, who is He? Someone I can run to for a 360-degree safe zone. Speaking of running, this brings us to our final destination of conception.

I may sound cliché, but I saved the best for last; and I have to admit, this one is my favorite, mostly due to its double meaning. In Latin, the word "recursion" translates into *recursio,* denoting a "running back to" or a "returning from."[5] We must consider that the initial step to birth as the Word of God is to return from the old ways you've known and run back to the Lord, who is the only Way. Allow Him to direct the channels in your mind, tweak the heat that you've suffered under, and reprune the branches that are unfruitful. Without God, you cannot beat this on your own. Human resources can only get you so far until you're back in the pit of defeat, not to mention the elephant that would live with you. There would be an emptiness in your soul that is always hungry for more, asking for a deeper meaning to life.

By formation, we crave the Word. We were made by Him, through Him, and for Him, to become Him. Who could better solve your identity cube than the One who shaped it? Who could better arrange your Jenga pieces without breaking you? He knows what triggers you and what excites you. He knows the genuine desires of your heart. When you run back home to God, you're running back for the keys. The missing pieces are planted in the location in which you were conceived. That's why a childhood home brings back memories, because your roots made you who you are today. Your roots authenticate your story. So go! Run backward. Rewind and find the Word in you. He's there somewhere. All you have to do is remove the dirt to see His fingerprints.

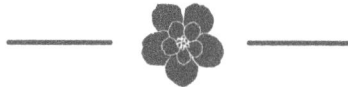

Recursio may have sparked a fire in your belly, but the English version is getting ready to take it home for you.

Recursion is a generating of the next number or result in a series by reapplying the algorithm on which the series is based, back to the number or result in the series that precede it.[6]

Let's unpack this definition in terms of Kingdom:

A **generating** is your purpose, pending. To generate means to arise or come about; to create, make, or produce.[7]

The **next number** equates to the very next move of God. Your new identity, hence why numbers are used for identification.

A **series** denotes the sequence of your life. It is mentioned when one thing happens after another. In the book of Amos, God says things will begin to happen so fast your head will swim, one thing fast on the heels of the other.[8] I call it the *holy domino effect*.

Reapplying has two powerful characterizations:[9]

1. To apply (an existing rule or principle) in a different context. For instance, the coat of glory is applied on top of the coat of mental illness.

2. To spread (a substance) on a surface again. When I searched this definition on Oxford, it had an example sentence that stated, "To reapply sunscreen hourly." Or in better words, the Lord will provide around-the-clock protection from the thing that was meant to burn you!

Algorithm. The *Freedom Formula* is an algorithm God uses to deliver His people. Freedom, when separated in half, creates the hyphenated word "free-dom." Simply put, God came to *free* us from the *dom*inion that Satan had over us after the Fall. He provided an escape plan through 2 Corinthians 5:17. If any woman be in Christ, she is a new creature. The old has passed, and the new has come.

The ***Freedom Formula*** states:

✝ The Cross ÷ The Resurrection = The Reinvention of the Woman

- In elementary terms, when Jesus died, depression died too. Because He is Life, He cancelled out every physical, spiritual, and mental yoke.

- The word "reinvention" in this formula is defined as the action or process by which something is changed so much that it appears to be entirely new.[10] This has been God's specialty since the beginning. He does His best work on things that are shattered. He has a doctoral degree in the major of new, with a flawless, eternal dissertation to match!

Back to the number takes us back to our very first Identifier, Immanuel Himself.

In the series that precede it is the breaking of the chains on Calvary.

When combining every kingdom bit of this text, we have come to form a new definition.

Recursion is the unlocking of a woman's purpose in which the coat of glory reforms her blood. She is freed from the chains of death and identified as a new creation in the Messiah. Her old has passed away, and her new life has begun. She is clothed from head to toe, washed from the inside out, and ready for the very next move of God.

This might have taken you for a spin, but -*ception* is no stranger to you. As a matter of fact, you've been living out that word for as long as you've been depressed, except you were under the rules of a different foe, *deception.* Deception occurs when the truth has been deleted. You see, Satan uses recursion on us as well. He hides your face from your true identity, applies the opposite version of your character, alienates you from God, and cancels out your happiness. He wants to destroy you because you are a triple threat. You have access to all three impartations of God. You are biologically attached to the One he hates. This makes it imperative for you to answer your calling. He's your only way out. He has the key of victory.

Give the Doctor permission to impregnate you. If you do, the Word will be conceived in you right now. He'll run His blood through your vessels and relabel the access points that are dormant. He'll intercept every attack meant to harm you and design a new starting point through a process known as *inception.* While doing so, He'll make you the *exception,* someone who was overlooked by people, just to be looked at by the Creator—set apart for divine use.

At this time, I invite you into the presence of the Almighty. It doesn't matter what your religion is, or whether or not you are religious. I want you to have a new relationship with Christ. Relationship is what He wants from us, not a religious act. I have learned more about Him from my own personal walk than I ever have in all of my years in the church. As a woman with an unfortunate past, I am proof that He will welcome you with open arms. He is a good Father who erases all of our troubles with a simple cry, "Daddy, I need You." That's it.

So, right now, wherever you are, close your eyes and focus your attention on making the best phone call of your life. Quiet your anxiety, and try your hardest to bring about peace. Stay there for as long as you need to. Then open your eyes to read this prayer aloud:

"Heavenly Father, I thank You for answering my call for help. I present to You my pure heart, asking for a hand in freedom. The battle in my mind is too great to be healed by man. I need Your authority, Your power, Your love, Your grace. Visit me, Lord, and rewire my core. Teach me to be You on this earth. Teach me to become the Activated Word. I believe Christ died for this pain, and I also believe He rose to give me life—a life of abundance, full of power and truth. I thank You in advance for liberation, and I ask that You make Your home in me. Produce a brand new creation in the belly of my being. In Your name, I pray. Amen."

ACT on this!

Do you feel a tad bit closer to God after reading this chapter? Did you know Him before now? If so, how would you describe your relationship with Jesus? If not, are you excited to grow this divine connection?

GOD ACTS AS A BLEACHING AGENT WHEN HE RESTORES YOU

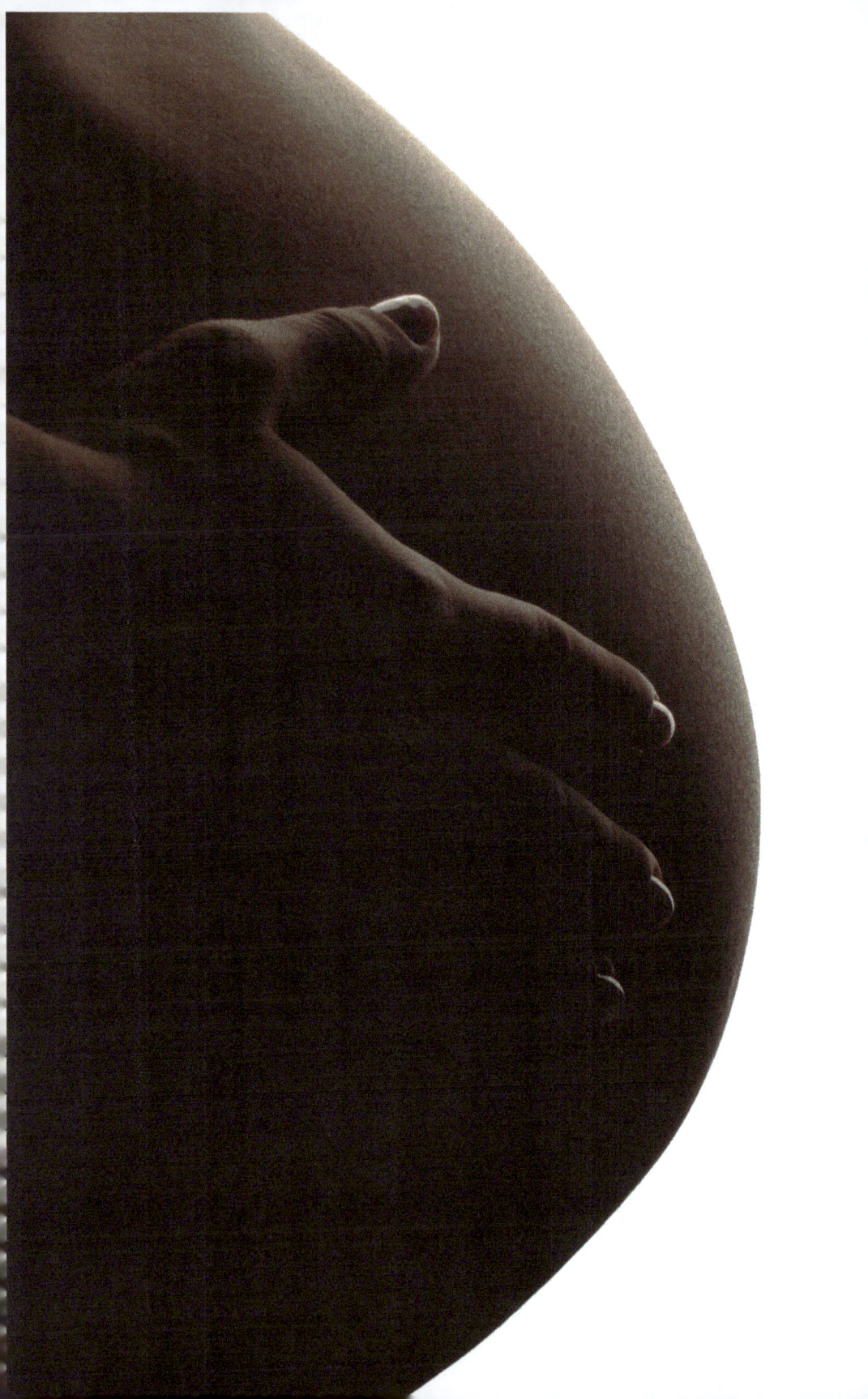

CHAPTER SIX

THE FIRST TRIMESTER

A New Creation

Once upon a time, there were Three. The Father, The Word, and the Holy Spirit. They activated as human flesh and birthed us into their bloodline. When the Enemy hit us with depression, that blood began to leak out until we fell into a deep state of unconsciousness. The Physician, God, diagnosed us of having Wordless disease. He then came up with a treatment plan to reactivate us. He fertilized our womb and embedded Himself as the key. A month after the procedure, we found out that we were pregnant with purpose. Now, we're overloaded with questions about what to expect on this new journey of becoming.

One of the very first apps a pregnant woman downloads on her phone is the BabyCenter app. This app prepares her for the changes her body will go through, the development of the baby, and the highs and lows of childbirth. It serves as the ultimate best friend for mommies to be, calming the many fears and doubts associated with creating new life. Birthing as the Word of God comes along with a similar platform. It's known as the SpiritCenter app. He will deposit this app in the center of your body, and you are to use it as a guidebook for transformation. Ran by the Holy Spirit, He only says and does what the Father permits. Holy Spirit tells you what to eat, how to speak, how to behave, which door to open and which to close. He does all of this while reassuring you what you mean to Him and how much He loves you. He is the all-inclusive, completely faithful Mate a girl could have.

The good news is that you've activated Him in the last chapter. He's searching the ways of your heart and the imbalances in your body. He's putting every structure back in position and gearing you up for birth.

The first trimester is the most critical phase. Baby develops rapidly, and Mommy feels a plethora of hormonal and physical ups and downs. With a new brain, heart, and spinal cord forming, the fetus is able to secure a base for the remainder of the pregnancy. He also sprouts inner organs, legs, arms, and budded fingers and toes. By the cessation of these 12 weeks, baby has reached approximately 3 inches long and is ready for the next three months of growth.

I remember being in this trimester with my daughter. I craved certain food and had revulsions to others where the thought of them would make me vomit. It's precisely how I felt when I began to swap mental illness for mental health. My mouth watered like a dog for the Word of God, and I could no longer eat nihilism. God was all that I wanted because He took the time to show me all that I was in Him. I began to study Scripture and find out where He mentioned me. As my appetite grew, my contagion sloughed away. I began to see a new brain taking shape, a new set of organs appearing, extremities budding forth. Within the first three months of my recovery, I gained a new identity. I was a depression survivor who was doing the impossible with the help of God alone! He was my rehab.

The Lord applied the *Freedom Formula* over my life in the combination of two closely related identifiers: the numbers three and nine. As we learned earlier, three is completion. However, nine also signifies completion...but with a twist. It's spiritually known as divine completion or finality, and it literally means, "That's enough." That's why Christ died at the ninth hour of the day, the reason for pregnancy being nine months long, and the explanation for the nine fruits of Holy Spirit.

Mental illness causes such a degradation in character that God needed to perfect each level of your getaway. Therefore, by referencing the 27 books of the New Testament, we'll receive a triple bundle of freedom. As we refer to the Scriptures, we'll equally divide the number of letters in the word "activated" to correlate each trimester, making it a total of nine letters that are grouped into threes. Each letter will also have three different subsections. For this period, let's begin your activation using the opening few: A, C, and T.

THE
Arrival

God knocks on the door of your heart three times. Each knock contains a stage that completes the advent triangle.

Stage 1: Saying YES unlocks the rest. Saying NO leaves you solo.

When God is ready to activate you as the Word, He'll announce Himself by an overwhelming presence of power. This is the kind of power that'll let you know He's still running the show. It sets off the advent, the arrival of Christ. He gently arrives in you by way of the Spirit, but He comes to make some noise, nevertheless. He comes to break apart your shell of resistance and confound the hardness of your psyche. At that moment, all sin is thrown out. Your flaws are erased, and your awareness of Him is heightened. He sends an army after you. He shows up for you and vibrates the atmosphere. You'll know He's here when you feel the butterflies in your stomach, the chills on your extremities, and tears welling up. You'll know it's

Him when you find yourself saying "yes" in your heart. "Yes, God! I will follow you. Lead me to the door of breakthrough."

Y.E.S. means to **Y**ield **E**xcellent **S**urrender. Yield, as in provide your all to Christ. This is the only word that will help you unlock the remaining stages of abundance. It's the code to the blood bank of all things, one that also welcomes the encryption: 937. If you look at your phone's keypad, you'll find that the letter Y is under the digit 9, divine completion and finality; the letter E is under the digit 3, completion and unity; and the letter S is under the digit 7, completion and perfection.

It is hardly surprising that alphabetically and numerically each of those identifiers birth completion. Obedience is the only road to release the maximum definition of God over sorrow.

Think about this.

If G.O.D. is the **G**estation **o**f **D**ivinity, then He is the ultimate Carrier of the supernatural. When you wish to unlock the supernatural, submission is the route you take. You will never be complete until you submit. "Yes" puts you in the game. "No" does just the opposite. N.O. **n**egates **o**pportunity and prevents the workings of the Spirit. "No" leaves you cold and naked in the middle of Antarctica.

Now, you may be curious as to why the Lord doesn't just make us do what He wants. He could do that, but is it not better to serve God because you want to? Versus Him forcing you? He is not One to strip us of free will. He's kind enough to give us a choice, a choice between the red pill or the blue. The red defines life exceedingly. The blue means life reduced. He simply offers you a plate. You can choose to eat of it or not. When you choose to take and eat, He'll make sure your cup spills over. You'll never want for anything. Your "yes" gives you a designated seat at every attraction of life without paying for it. God says this one's on Him. This pass was compensated in full by the Blood from the bank. Your only instruction here is to accept His hand.

How do you do that? First, you support the notion that nothing can be done without God. Second, you grasp that He never has and never will steer you in the wrong direction. Last, you let go. Let go of puppeteering your timeline, and give God the strings, for the edge of His cloak is both indestructible and inexhaustible. (see Mark 6:56)

Stage 2: He Cleans the Unseen.

Before I got pregnant with Josiah, I was on a type of birth control that gave me ovarian cysts. The cysts ruptured during the first few weeks of my pregnancy, causing violent cramps. It was like the baby saw the inner risk factors that could raise an eyebrow, and he killed them off. He cleansed me of the things I could not physically see for myself, quite resembling the Spirit of Sanitization.

God acts as a bleaching agent when He restores you. He searches the veins of your heart and any bacteria bathing in your chambers. He looks far and wide for the spores that may have seeped in after the final draft of your creation day. He buffs your home from top to bottom, dusting the ceilings of your mind, washing the windows of your senses, and polishing the floorboards of your direction. He gathers the wheat, the glorifiable, into a safe.

Then He burns the chaff, the abominable, in a lake of fire. (see Luke 3:17) This wise separation doesn't always come in an envelope that you would expect, though.

Many times, you'll be put in circumstances that look nothing like God, then find out later that it was Him the whole time. He has a mysterious way of cleaning you up. The Lord targets your struggle and the aggravating ticks that have indented your flesh. He sweeps everything:

The unpleasant emotions.

The unforgiveness.

The obsessions, and so forth.

As deep as the germs go, He goes even further to locate the strains and pluck them out, making sure that He can fit. A baby could not survive in a dirty womb. Neither could the Word mature in filth. One or the other must go. In this regard, it is the dirt that leaves. Your health stays put. Your deliverance continues on. Your name carries on. Don't rebuke the cleaning process. Learn to embrace it.

Stage 3: A Kingdom-Made Blockade

At the close of seven weeks in utero, the mucus plug develops. This corkscrew protects the womb from infection. With this blockade, baby is kept harm-free. Nothing can enter. Nothing can leak out. Over the course of nine months, this cork becomes the head security guard for the fetus. It stands watch for anything that attempts to trespass the borderline, and it will use the heaviest machinery, if need be, to shelter the baby.

Retrieval of the Word involves the same tendencies. Kingdom has its very own military team of defense. With the mission to safeguard your rebirth, Holy Spirit will choose His top seven generals to oversee your case: Joy, Strength, Peace, Love, Trust, Wisdom, and Grace. Each are highly skilled and respected in their field of training.

General one, Joy. She's the day-maker. Joy meets you in the mornings with a beautiful stack of pancakes and an itinerary of events to keep you busy rejoicing. She loves to ease your mental breakdowns with a well of contentment. General two, Strength. She's your robotic twin. Strength is you without the fear and weakness buttons. With her, there is nothing you cannot do. General three, Peace. She is a serial killer. Confusion and panic won't stand a chance against her bullets that surpass all understanding. General four, Love. She wears the always crystal around her neck. Love always protects, always trusts, always hopes, and always perseveres. General five, Trust. She's your platinum card. When you swipe her, the Lord labels your pathway with the inside of His hands. He designs a route without the traffic, accidents, or tolls. Even in the dark, you'll never have trouble finding clarity. General six, Wisdom. She is a stunning woman. Wisdom is worth far more than rubies, yet easier to come by. The Spirit releases Wisdom as an insurance policy. She's mastered the heart and mind of God. If your thoughts are warped, she repairs them. If your actions are thrown out of whack, she mends them. Whatever needs fixing, she fixes.

Then there's Grace, general seven. Meet the spiritual G.O.A.T.

of the team. Her sufficient influence makes her the greatest of all time. She's the filling. The muscles and bones of the body. The neuronal connections of the brain. The healer of flesh-inflicted thorns. The power perfecter. When God says His grace is enough, believe Him. Grace covers inability with the phrase, "I am able." She sparkles in the can-dos of the Lord. In her presence, you can, and you will. In her absence, you won't make it past the front door.

These seven defenders form a blockade in your womb. They shelter the growth of God, while roasting diabolical infection.

THE
Confidant

He takes the heat by rescuing you from three central fires of emotional arrest. Each time He acts as your Extinguisher, He serves on a new level of unity with you.

Primary Level: Your Vault by Default

Commonly, you find people stashing away their prized possessions. From a young age, we've learned to keep diaries, lockets, love notes, favorite photos, and boyfriend's letterman jackets hidden in special places. If anyone dared to touch our things, we would threaten to harm them. I have younger siblings. I know how inquisitive they can be.

Though I don't believe any of us would really commit a crime over a diary, I trust that it was more about the vulnerability that our possessions held. If my diary was read aloud, I'd be trapped in that common nightmare, the one where you're standing naked on a stage, and there's a crowd of people staring at you. I would've been mortified if my secrets were released. Everyone would know my problems. My mistakes. My fears.

I think a lot of us remain in that grade-school way of thinking, even as we come to know the Lord. We figure if we state our issues, wrongdoings, and inner thoughts out loud to Him, we'll become a target. We are so afraid of His judgement that we often forget His love means the most.

Let me ask you something: When you were keeping secrets back then, guess who knew about them? When you began fighting depression, guess who knew about it and loved you through it? Humiliation is the farthest from God's embrace. He doesn't want you to feel ashamed or embarrassed when you come to Him. He just wants you to come. By default, He is thrilled to be your vault of emotional keepings.

Your call for help moves God with compassion! He says to give everything to Him, and He can take it. His yoke is easy, and His burden is light. From the wretched self-hate to the adopted fear from your past, He wants it all. Your secrets are safe with Him. God will privately deal with you, so He can publicly show your winning season.

Secondary Level: A Father to a Toddler

Fathers are the identity-givers of the parental match. These men are gifted with influence they don't even realize. Your relationship with your father reflects your relationship with yourself. If your mother tells you that you are beautiful and talented, you'll sort of brush it off as if it was something that she was supposed to say. If your father tells you the same thing, you'll savor those words. There would be invisible markings of those identities written all over your body.

A solid paternal relationship is a self-esteem booster. I always wished I had been lucky enough to be a girl who could jump into Daddy's arms while he whispered greatness in my ears. Unfortunately, my relationship with my dad was stolen from me. He did his best to financially provide, but he missed out on the biggest parts of my life: my character, my traits, my personality, me.

A myriad of sons and daughters around the globe have wrestled just the same, if not worse. We were robbed of those diamonds that are only formed with one's father. Continuing on, the lack of material seed carries over into our relationship with our Creator Dad. We cuff Him to this bracket that says, "If my dad left, God will leave me also." We never give Him a fighting chance to prove His word. We disqualify Him before He approaches the plate to bat the ball. How unfair is that, to limit His potential to our own subjective experience?

There are primitive and secure grounds on which He stands as the Father. God's protection is more effective than any human's.

Regardless of our age, He sees us as toddlers learning to walk and talk. Each area of growth is a learning curve that grows our faith.

My first son taught me a lesson when he progressed from standing to walking. I saw him fall on his hands and knees a truckload of times before he got the hang of it. He never once gave in the towel. If anything, he worked harder because he could smell how close he was to the finish line. What a joy this was for me, being available to support my child in both his failures and accomplishments. All I needed to do was guide him until he could handle himself, and I remained close by when He needed Mommy.

God works the same in you. He supports you when it seems like you're carrying more weight than you can manage, for He knows the strength that will emanate from the trial period. He guides you, watches you stumble, picks you back up, and shoots you directly into triumph. Once the training wheels are removed, He pulls out the first aid kit, ready to bandage you up for the next test of faith. He will never leave your side during this time, and He'll always lend His chest for your cries. He turns out to be the Father you cannot live without.

Tertiary Level: A Friend who Comprehends

The Lord's application for the role of Best Friend is background-proof worthy. Christ dealt with rejection from His own kind, denial from one of His closest friends, and backstabbing from another. He faced every type of mental illness, persecution, and brutalization there is. "He Himself, took our infirmities and bore our sickness." (Matthew 8:17) He knows what it feels like to suffer, which is why

He's capable of empathizing with you.

A true friendship involves two people who value each other above themselves. They confide in one another and trust each other through thick and thin. A best friend might be closer to you than your own spouse. You can be your truest self around this person without ever affecting the intimacy of the relationship. They love you for who you are, and you love them no less. The both of you will do whatever it takes to stay tight.

I discovered a best friend in the Word during my transition. I spent the majority of my days confiding in Him, and He listened and replied on the spot. A friendship with the Lord is not under-leveled compared to a physical friendship. He speaks your language, He hears your concerns, and He feels your anxiety. He sees you.

God is a Crosswalk. He's the type who will put you on a lift, free from agony, while He places your burdens on His back and climbs Mount Everest. Unlike the undependable nature of man, He imparts the highest level of companionship available. When you feel the urge to pick up your phone to text or call a friend about something that's bothering you, try Him first. He'll listen, He'll understand, and He just might shock you.

THE
Teacher

Studying all things Word is organized in three realms of education: primary, secondary, and university. As it is in education, let it be complete in the Kingdom that grows in you.

Primary: Eat the Pages in Stages

Rabbi, Master, Professor, Teacher! God fulfills each of these roles. He's taken the prerequisites for the long line of degrees He's achieved. He's aced Life 101, Spiritual Education, Eternal History, Struggle Studies, and Kingdom Arts. He's been approved so that He could teach you how to follow His lead. He is fluent in preparation, dedication, and vigor. He's bursting in wisdom, knowledge, and personal adventure. No one knows Scripture better than the Word of God Himself. And the beautiful thing about Him being all that He is, is that He lives in you. That means you have grand access to the Teacher's Manual.

The force of God is driven through His people. But if you're operating His vehicle on E, then your mode of transportation will be towed off the side of the road. What good is it to go to a dealership, purchase a Bugatti, and never feed it fuel? No matter how valuable something is, if it lacks fuel, it lacks movement.

Let us apply this same rule to getting pregnant with your new identity. Without feeding your spirit with the Bible, your purpose will be malnourished, and there's a reason for that.

In a human pregnancy, the unborn fetus is attached to the umbilical cord, which attaches to the placenta, which is latched onto the inside of the mother's uterus. In your supernatural pregnancy, the unborn fruit is your new creation as the Word, the placenta is the Father and Son duo, and the umbilical cord is Holy Spirit. They are architecturally interwoven in you.

Now, let's swim a little deeper than that.

An umbilical cord has three vessels that help to nourish the child: two arteries that carry waste away from the baby, and one vein that carries oxygen and nutrients back to the baby. In your case, the Father and Son are the two Arteries that cleanse your spirit, while the Holy Vein feeds your evolution. The Trinity empowers you to give into that which is growing in your belly. This is why failing to eat the Breath of God places you at risk for a miscarriage, or worse, birthing the Word with defects. Just as a baby can die from starvation in the womb, so can your new identity. Eating the Pages, however, will protect against these risks. They will provide the energy needed for your activation.

As soon as Jesus revealed Himself to me, He got me started on the Word diet. I absorbed the Scriptures as food, and they gave me fuel. He met me at my dining room table for the next three months, while I prepped for my calling. He prescribed me an enhancing medication, something known as the "who/why" pills. These were the perfect tablets for seeing Him in a different, yet brighter light than before. This drug is advised for people who have departed from His presence, those who need a wider expanse of knowledge and wisdom, and for those who are new carriers of the Word. Side effects include healthier thoughts and clearer vision.

The who/why pill answers two dominant questions:

1. Who is the Word of God? (Who are we in Him, and who is He in us?)

2. Why did He put on an outfit of flesh?

The quickest and most effective way for you to be born of God is to gain a comprehensive standard on who He is and why He came. The books of the Bible will show you that He died to release you from the curse of the law, to offer you grace and truth—gifts that were only made available through His sacrifice. By standing in the gap between you and the Father, Christ carried your tribulations with Him to the Cross. He bore the weight of your pain and defeated death for you. The only thing He wants in return is for you to become the best version of yourself.

By formation, we have a burning fire for the Word of God. It is our earthly experiences that hide the Father's profile. So, in order to reveal that news again, we'd have to get to know Him. Doing this will open up a portal so strong that we won't have to go searching to find ourselves in the world.

Jesus assigned me the New Testament when I began my study sessions. This was not a happy accident. It was a movement. The word "testament" signifies a cause or a belief, thereby leaving the Old to be filled with outdated beliefs and the New to serve as the apostolical, updated version of the Word—tweaked and reinvented to equal Kingdom ethics. Beginning in John, I was educated on the truest origin of God.

John presents Christ as the Preliminary Activated Word:
"In the beginning was the Word, and the Word was with God, and the Word was God. He was in the beginning with God. All things were made through Him, and without Him nothing was made that was made." (John 1:1-3)

The Breath of Man:
"In Him was life, and the life was the light of men." (John 1:4)

The Brilliance of Void:
"And the light shines in the darkness, and the darkness did not comprehend it." (John 1:5)
"…the True Light which gives light to every man coming into the world." (John 1:9)

The Reciprocated Grace:
"…of His fullness we have all received, and grace for grace." (John 1:16)

The Glory Carrier:
"…and we beheld His glory, the glory as of the only begotten of the Father, full of grace and truth." (John 1:14)

The Granter of Holy Spirit:
"…this is He who baptizes with the Holy Spirit." (John 1:33)

After John, remain in the Gospels and continue on with Matthew's definition of the chosen people. Matthew spends an ample amount of time proving our identities.

We are the elements that fuel the earth:
"You are the salt of the earth…" and "… the light of the world." (see Matthew 5:13-14)

We are the fortunate children of a present Father figure:
"If you then…know how to give good gifts to your children, how much more will your Father in heaven give good things to those who ask Him!" (Matthew 7:11)

After Matthew, move on to Mark and Luke. They further show Christ walking as a Life Guru, Universal Donor, Chief of Surgery, and Power Source. This is indicated by His teachings of the Gospel, His healing hand, and the divine miracles He performed. The Lord's library of novels here were so extensive that the world itself could not hold the number of books that would be written about Him.

The Book of Acts identifies believers as the **Act**ivated Word. I take it as no coincidence that the book, which is titled Acts, is the initial release of Holy Spirit who activates us as God. We were inactive up until the apostles received the Spirit in the Upper Room. Without Him, we could only perform the supernatural under a cap. With Him, we were given gifts without limits. Acts 2:17 writes, *"In the last days, says God, I will pour out My Spirit on all flesh. Your sons and daughters will prophesy, your young men will see visions, your old men will dream dreams."*

Romans through Jude profess the remainder of the Holy Handbook in terms of manifesting as Christ:

"…receive with meekness the implanted word, which is able to save your souls. Be doers of the word, and not hearers only, deceiving yourselves. For if anyone is a hearer of the word and not a doer, he is like a man observing his natural face in a mirror; for he observes himself, goes away, and immediately forgets what kind of man he was." (James 1:21-24)

Revelation is the end of times. This book has the secrets of the unseen world, and the events of the future. The word "future" is used lightly here, for I am certain that we are presently living in Revelation. The apocalypse is all around us. We just have to look beyond the world and into Heaven. That's where the crown of life is.

After studying the New Testament, make your way to the beginning of Scripture and get acquainted with the last portion of this method, your "why." The Old Testament is a collection of beautiful stories that foretell the reason God dropped in on us, that which taught us how to morph into the fullness of Him.

As you nurse on the Milk, I recommend reading three chapters per day. Anything more, and the information may not stick. Anything less, and you may slow down your progress. Keep in mind that these words were written for you. You are the Pages of Life. He needs you to passionately bite the verses as if you were eating your favorite food. Envision the Bible as your pizza, tacos, Chinese, or apple pie. The moment you sit down to read should be the moment you smell your desired meal. Drool over the Word.

Consume the Word. Befit the Word. This is your power. Use it!

Focus on understanding by engaging in active reading and notetaking daily. Dedicate a notebook, binder, folder, or notes on your phone to Word study. Include the verses that pop out to you, any revelation He gives you, and the summary of each chapter in your own words.

It also helps to buy a study Bible with commentaries. If you cannot afford to grab one, search online for the divine messages that other believers have gotten from the same readings. Under no circumstance, however, should you use the commentaries as the foundation of retrieval. They're just the extras. What you personally receive is what will heal you best. Never neglect the impartation that God speaks to you directly. He teaches a unique sense of His Breath in every one of His children's hearts. Find out what He's saying to you.

Aside from that, look at your deliverance as a thrilling pursuit, not a dull one! Feel free to color-code and organize your notes in any custom that inspires you. See into the Bible as you would a television or a social media feed. Your dedication to read will serve you well.

It is a full-course meal for anyone who will believe and receive. In it are the words of life, and without it are the holes of death. Eat and be filled with the Eternal Word of God.

Secondary Education: Communication Equals Relation

Prayer is a dreaded topic. Some people never pray because they do not understand what prayer actually is. But it's much simpler than you think. First of all, there are no rules. When Christ taught us how to pray in Luke 11, He provided a guideline to help lead us into prayer. He did not force us to pray in one particular manner or another. He highlighted the skill of conversation.

When you speak with a person, you greet one another ("Hey Olivia, nice to see you!"), you speak what's on your mind (including anything that you're excited or worried about), you make plans, advice might be given, and goodbyes are said. Prayer is no different. When you pray, you greet the Lord ("Heavenly father, God, Christ, etc.), you express your feelings or current issues ("I'm having some trouble at work…"), you ask Him for guidance ("Can You strengthen me for this interview?"), you thank Him for what He's doing in your life, and you say your goodbyes ("Amen").

The twist here is that a talk with God is more efficient than a talk between humans. He knows you best, He hears you best, and He has a vehicle of resources catered to your appeal. Still, it's just a conversation. Prayer is defined as speaking to God because it produces an action. The suffix -er means to act upon.[1] So in pray-er, you're acting upon the heart of God. You're getting His attention.

Piggybacking off of this, the Greek word for "pray" is proseuchomai,[2] which is an interaction between you and the Father that replaces your will for His. Thus, you act upon His heart, and you likely adapt His ways. That's why Jesus says, "Yet not My will, but Yours be done." (Luke 22:42 NIV)

Speaking with God helps to build a sturdy relationship between the two of you, as it does in any relationship. Prayer is just an elevated talk that fills in the gaps of your soul. Stay mindful of that, and it will feel more like an honor to pray, versus an obligation laced with rules. Some might ask, "What's the purpose of prayer if God already knows our needs?" The answer is that when you come to Him with a heart of expectancy, ready to receive His blessings, you loosen the knots in your mind. It's the key to absolute peace. Also, whatever you're asking for could be found in the prayer itself. Several believers have testified that our answers are buried in the dialogue with Heaven. God shoots down answers as we fly up our requests. Many times, He's responded to me before I had the chance to end my prayers. If that's not incredible, I don't know what is.

Whether you prefer to pray in your thoughts, out loud, in the shower, in your car, or in your closet, talk to Jesus in a way that helps you feel relaxed. He knows your heart and will be pleased to hear from you. Desire a prayer-powered life. It doesn't cost you anything but a few minutes of your time, and the effects are powerful. Prayer delivers. Prayer is the cure. Prayer is your armor. Put it on.

College Education: Audibility Releases Security

The ear is the most obedient feature of the human body. The mouth is the most rebellious. We spend all day talking and not enough time listening. This becomes a ritual of poisoned insecurity.

People are so busy running their mouths that I'm pretty sure they would overlook news reports of the earth spinning off its axis. What a deaf world we live in, so caught up in the pants of the mouth that we never give our ear any play. One lesson I've learned from the Mastermind is to be quick to listen and slow to speak. (James 1:19 NIV) That means 90 percent of the day should be dedicated to the ear, while only 10 percent should be given into words. I used to resent myself for being the outcast in every discussion. Never having anything to add, not interested in the chosen topic, and keeping my silence instead, constantly wondering, *What is wrong with me? Why do I have such a hard time fitting in?*

It wasn't until the Spirit reminded me of His personal technique that I was able to see things differently. Christ was a natural listener. If you really study His image, you'll find that He spent the majority of His time heeding conversation before leading it. He acquired the ear to hear from childhood. When He was a young boy, His family lost Him for three days. After knocking on doors and backtracking their steps, they found that little Jesus had been in the temple the whole time, observing and listening to the instructors.

I want you to catch something here.

He is God. He knew the hearts of all, even at this age. But He decided to use His physical ear over His spiritual knowledge. When He called the people out on their messy behavior, He used human recall in place of His godly senses. The Messiah's three-and-a-half-year ministry is a fine example of this. His sermons consisted of what He'd physically heard for 30 years.

The corrupt mindsets.

The immorality.

The lawlessness.

He spent almost 90 percent of His life listening to the poison, before educating a single thing. We were taught a valuable lesson in His mouthguard: how to activate our audibility.

The Lord paid attention to the words of man and to the words from the Father. He learned how to measure what people believed, in contrary to God's will for them. He received direction, nuggets of wisdom, updates about His calling, and empowerment. It was all downloaded directly to His ear. If He had been too busy speaking, the sacrifice would be untouched. Something so great would've been impossible for Him to tackle without instruction. His audible agreement secured Him.

My question to you is this: Are you ready for that same security? The reading and the praying hold no value if you're narrow-sensed. Practice hearing the voice of God. Start with about five minutes a day writing down what the Lord is saying to you. You'll know He's speaking when you feel a positive urge or a leap in your stomach. Often, He'll give you an epiphany about yourself, Him, or the world. You may find yourself saying, "Wow, I never realized that," or, "That's an interesting way to look at it."

Learn to be receptive throughout the day. Stay ready for the current events. God is a reliable God who never misses a beat. He's forever streaming His voice. We just need to tune in.

ACT *on this!*

Reading the Bible is such a daunting task when we try to read it like a regular book. That's the number one reason we fail at it. It cannot be compared to a published manuscript because it's not just a book. It's *the* Book. Scripture is the fundamental code of mankind. There is a message to be received in all 1,189 chapters of it. After reading "Eat the Pages in Stages," are you more confident to study the Word of God? How will you fit it into your schedule?

YOUR DESIGN IS LIKE DIVERTICULITIS TO THE SATANIC ESTATE

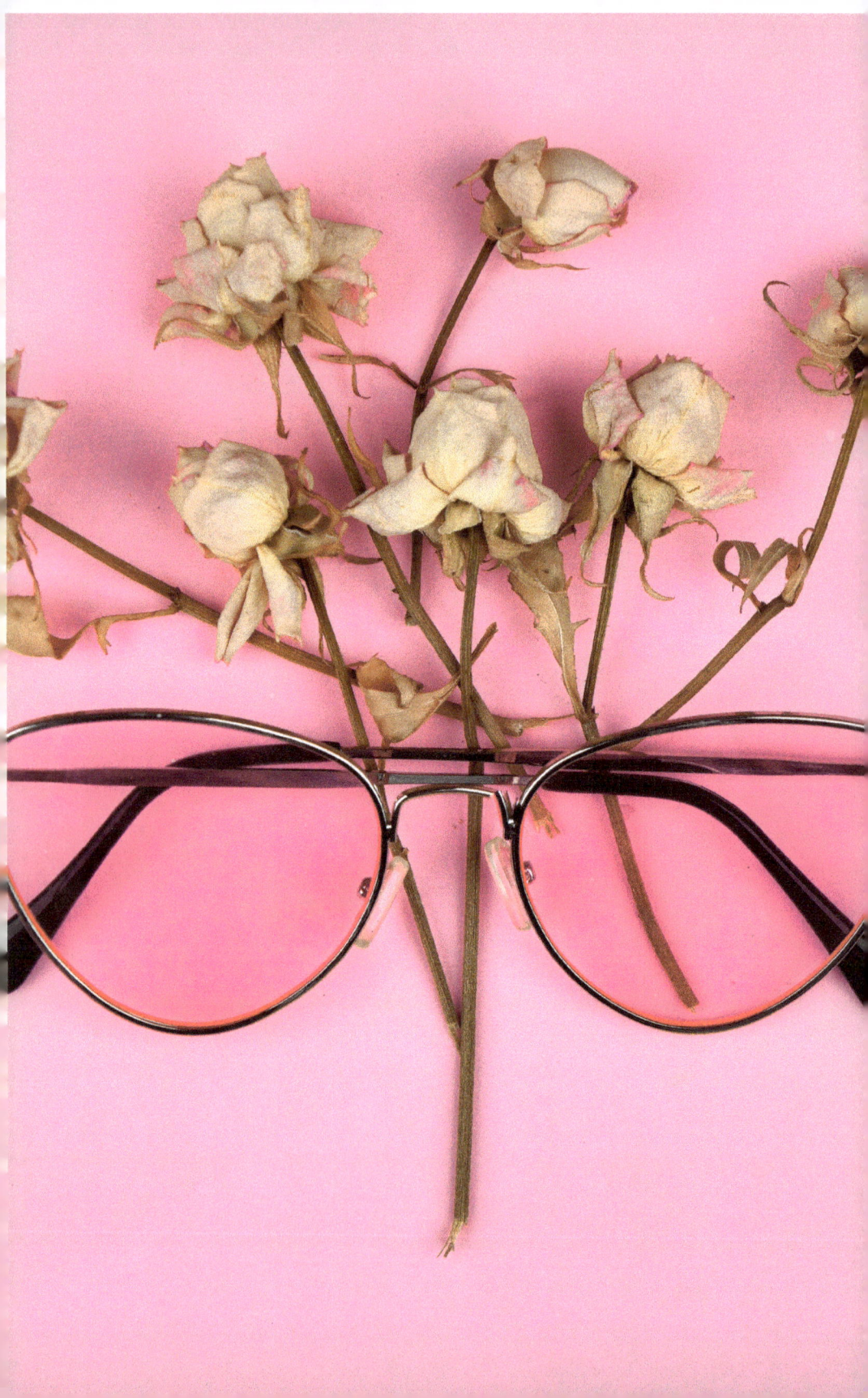

CHAPTER SEVEN

THE SECOND TRIMESTER

A Rose-Colored Lens

For most mothers, the second trimester is the easiest of the three. Nausea and vomiting have subsided by now, and you're not yet dealing with the swollen feet and shortness of breath. This is the time you're able to really enjoy your new baby bump. Some would say this period brings out the rose-colored glasses. Going shopping for the nursery, finding out the gender of the baby, and finally revealing the news to family and friends are some things a mother-to-be looks forward to. The most critical phase of development has elapsed, and you're able to visualize the bright lights ahead of you.

I was stunned to witness myself going from a place of dusk, where all I could see were the pits of Hell, to a heavenly abode of endless possibilities concerning my future. When I would hear failure beginning to rise, the Lord would hastily remind me of my worth. He showed me who I was, what I was capable of, and what He had given me the keys to. He brought me on the rollercoaster of reality, using the next set of letters of activated: I, V, and A.

THE
Identity

God renames you on three major forms of identification: your birth certificate, your driver's license, and your social security card.

Birth Certificate: A Creation for the Nations

I believe every one of us has a manuscript to author. We all have a story to tell. That's the reason our Creator hosts each of our names and stories in the heavenly books. We have all been through something that is worth recording. If it is useful in Heaven, surely it is useful here. We should treasure our testimonies and offer them on a silver platter as dipping sauce. Millions of people need to hear from you. Nations await your reinvention. Rooms, mountain tops, and time zones have your name on them. Cities need to be conditioned. States are on standby. Countries are idle. The purpose in you activates the wind of it all. Your inner adversity is someone else's victory. If you believe that God was just going to throw away the evidence of your hardship, I'm here to abolish that thought right now. God uses everything! If you've been through it, He can use it.

Nothing is held back from the total release of God's glory over your life. You've survived it to help another thrive from it. Satan fought his hardest to prevent your possession of the Word. He knew the moment you conceived you will have escaped his throne and opened up a torrent of miracles that cannot be shut down or glitched under any circumstance. Your wisest, wealthiest, and healthiest decades are closer than you think. Mental illness has made you an impervious force. Now, there is nothing blocking you.

Frankly, was there ever? Your birth was a blessing to us all. Your design is like diverticulitis to the satanic estate. The outer layer of your body contains a gold-plated suit. Your fingers are drowning in gold dust. Your hair is aurum-colored. Your feet are wrapped in a satin gold. Your eyes are lined in liquid amber. Your lips are painted with a golden tint. You are an heir of a chosen, royal priesthood. (1 Peter 2:9) You are God's special possession. *That* is who you are.

An irreplaceable fossil that the world is famished for.

The echo of His identity.

Driver's License: Qualities over Wannabes

I drained my life trying to change the person that I am. Pleasing others used to be my motivation. I brightened the few great qualities that I had, and I hated the flaws that overshadowed the good. You're unaware of your faults until people start calling them out. By the time they're finished identifying what's wrong with you, you doubt there's anything decent left. I've endured the persecutions. I know how confused a woman can be when she's trying to find herself on the world's stage. Being under those flames has caused me to reimagine my personality. I used to be the type who would go home and mentally slice off every rotten element that had been spoken against me that day. I cut off masses of myself for the approval of people. But thanks to God, not everything went down the drain.

I've been blessed to hold on to a few unique qualities along the way, those that make me a dynamite today. For instance, I've always been passionate, one who is so tenacious and nonconforming that I often shouted my point across in a debate. My intentions weren't to yell, just to explain it the best way I knew how. Many times, I failed to notice my voice ascending to the roof and my hands dancing to the syllables of my words. Yet even in my sincerity, this flaw was used as ammo against my self-esteem. I abhorred this quality of mine, and sought to fix it my whole life to please people. But the Lord spoke to me one day regarding my viewpoint. He said, "What you have identified as flaws all this time, have actually been hidden gifts that needed to be trained."

He wanted me to live out Romans 12:2, not to conform to

the pattern of this world, but to be transformed by the renewing of my mind. The passion was never a fault to begin with. It was a gift from God to empower my calling. Had I not been born with a fervent spirit, my holy stance would be diluted. How would I fight against the forces of darkness without an insane amount of determination? How could I have sat down and written this story without a strong desire to help my reader? The fight has never been easy, and I'm sure it never will be, but the finish line has been reachable because of my passion. God did not have to coach me on how to stand for what I believed in. He just had to show me when it was appropriate to release it and how much of it to use. He trained my faults as contributions for Kingdom.

He wants to do this in all of us if we let Him. You do not have to accept your flaws as flaws. See them as hidden gifts. Your time here is too short to waste it wishing you were one way or the other. You should spend your days watering the organic qualities, instead of letting others dehydrate them. The Lord has given *you* the license to drive. Your flaws are *yours* to grow into something special, not anyone else's. And the second you start to beat yourself up about a flaw, think about getting pulled over for steering in the wrong direction, gaining one point against your license every time you want to become something you're not.

Learn to accept the unaccepted about yourself. Stand up for you when no one else will. Be your biggest defender. We have too many wannabes already.

Act different than them!

Don't be afraid to love yourself!

On these merits, I have a short activity I would like to share with you, one that helped me identify my hidden gifts. Grab a sheet of paper and something to write with. At the top of the paper title it "A License to Drive." Then draw a three-columned chart that fills the remainder of the sheet. Let's call the first column "Alleged Flaw." In this column, write a list of flaws that you have accepted all these years. Title the next column "Root Cause." Take a ride down memory lane, and try to remember what you believe may have caused the flaw. Feel free to write "inbred" if you carried it with you in the womb. Title the last column "Hidden Gift." Use this space to conjure up the benefits that could birth from what you thought was an identity stain. For example, if one of my flaws was jealousy, I would state that becoming the best version of me would prevent envy. Jealousy could be driven into willpower—used for a greater purpose in my achievements, rather than fired against my sister in Christ.

As you identify your faults, think of the activity as brain dumping your issues onto the table and sorting them out into a giftbox. You're identifying gifts that you can bring with you wherever you go, gifts to bless the world with.

Social Security Card: Your Look Is a Closed Book
In our culture, if you have lips like Kylie, hips like Beyoncé, boobs like Kate Upton, and blemish-free, baby soft skin, congratulations! You are officially the quintessential woman. Deduct any one of those markers, and you're as ugly as the creatures on the ground. No wonder females are at a high risk for developing mental illness.

If we're not the Barbie type, we're not enough. Body precision is impossible to keep up with. Why did we ever hand over our security to the social world? How did this happen? Where does this stem from? Who gave them rights over our bodies? Society has made us an open book of typos, grammatical slips, and punctuation errors. It tells us that we are not worthy of their morals. We don't fit the benchmark to be published in the archives of beauty.

Women are pieces of Play-Doh here. We are precast and shaved into a typical look. We are made to copy appearances, generally in an unrealistic version of a human. Doesn't that sound like plagiarism to you? When did fake ever become the definition of gorgeous? When did altering your physiognomies become the perfect replacement for your natural? They've burned our eyes out. Real means phony nowadays, and it's sickening to never be able to differentiate between the two.

I often see magazines that are headlined, *The most beautiful woman in the world*, basically encouraging us to spend our last penny on shaping ourselves into her. What twisted mortal came up with that foolishness? Who are they to decide who the most attractive person on the planet is? Are there certain qualifications that need to be met, and aren't these models bathing in a plastic casing anyhow? This is a bizarre game of cat and mouse. Society is a god, and we are its followers. We are committed to a system that doesn't even love us, a system that wants to change us, a system that sends us into a mental plague.

I had a vision about this once. I saw a town filled with people who were downcast and rejected. They were carrying old, dirty books that were stapled to their chests. Ripped out were pages lying on the ground that were burned around the edges. These were the scripts of sacrifice. People were giving up their genuine biology for artificiality. I later saw the Lord collecting their true identities, gracefully walking through the town, picking up the missing pages, and placing them back into each person's book. As He added them, the pages suddenly turned a candy apple red, and the books were redeveloped. His warmth kindled their unfading features. Those He helped became new creations that day. They'd found their happiness not in the world, but in the love of God. Because He called them perfect, they believed it. Because He said their look was a closed book, they ran with it.

I used to be the woman with pages lying about. Two years ago, you wouldn't have caught me in public without a full face of makeup. I reviled my face and body. I let the social organisms rule me. I listened to their anti-affirmative quotes, wondering if people treated me badly because of my looks. I had an awful viewpoint of attraction. With eyebrows drawn on, lips overlined, eyeliner reaching my temples, bronzer packed on deep, and concealer bright under my eyes, I probably looked like a vampire beauty queen. I learned the ritualistic way of applying makeup, soon realizing that their methods weren't to enhance my features, but to erase them. They played me until God saved me. He unraveled my undone. He showed me the backside of skin-deep—that beauty is actually soul-deep.

The Bible says that a real ornament is someone who revitalizes her inner self, someone with a gentle, quiet spirit. He refers to that woman as His greatest value, a rare diamond. He teaches her to proudly assume her nudity, encouraging her to focus more on skincare instead of skin manipulation…not to ban her from wearing makeup, but to inspire her to fall in love with the underneath.

He's talking to you today. Break loose from the chains hooked to the standards. Find the loveliest you. Become confident in your bare skin before you apply that first drop of foundation. You cannot be controlled if *the* Foundation is your number one fan. Your look is filled with the glory of the Lord. (2 Corinthians 3:18)

You are a seamless, hard-covered novel with red pages. You are innately stunning! Own your natural, girl.

THE *Vision*

God premieres your future, using three different types of visual awareness, starting with the most reliable and ending with the least.

20/20: Imagine what could happen if you were to eliminate the what ifs. Imagine if fear wasn't an emotion here. Imagine if there were no limits, if someone offered to invest in your wildest dreams, if you knew for a fact that you could not lose. What would you do, knowing that anything was possible? What would you go after? Who would you become? As humans, we feel everything. We see the world as it is. There's only a small ratio of us who actually fulfill our heart's desire, a whopping 8 percent to be exact.[1] The rest of us are too busy watching for the possible hazards.

The rejection: What if I'm turned down?

The fallbacks: What if I make a mistake along the way?

The absent toolset: What if I'm not enough?

Distractions are so loud that we never look to the One who's highly familiar with it all. The One who sees the trenches before we do. The One who bargains to be our Tour Guide. As we see it all too clearly, we cannot see things clearly. Perfect vision is the polar opposite of perfect faith. Due to the what ifs, we never dare to dream about the absolutes. Truth that can only be shown through the lenses of the Spirit. 20/20 vision might be a good thing on earth, but it's an abomination to divine awareness. When you rely more on the flesh to guide you, you impede the help from your GPS—your Godly Positioning System.

The road to Damascus preaches loudly on this matter. Paul was very familiar with the changes in vision and how they determine your final chapters. Once a believer in persecuting God, next a believer in persecuting the Enemy with an iron fist, he was proof that "a person without vision is unrestrained." (Proverbs 29:18) The Lord performed eye surgery on Paul in three phases: the phase of 20/20, in which He baptized him in astonishment of His glory; the phase of 20/70, where He called him out by name and set him apart; and the phase of 20/200, where He drove him toward the Gospel. Like Paul, we are sent through the same three phases before our faith-walk pleases God. We advance from Godless vision to Godly imagination during our first appointment with Him. Similar to corrective surgery, He gets your feet wet in excitement by showing you the x-rays of how you'll look once He's finished working on you.

Consider this stage as the animated movie *Meet the Robinsons*. Lewis, the lead character in that film, meets disappointment in the middle of a project he had been singing praises about. The frustration causes him to throw away his destiny. He finds himself fighting against the "what if" demons in his mind:

"What if I'm not called to be an inventor? What if I'm just wasting time and energy on something I'll never really achieve?"

At the brink of losing the war, something awe-striking happens to him. Lewis gets the opportunity to envision his future with a beautiful family and a career as the richest inventor of his time. After this experience, he gains a laser-focused attitude. He holds to the fact that no matter what may come his way, God has shown him that he wins in the end. The mountains cannot squeeze him to death. The failures won't know his name. The mistakes will energize his game. Lewis's vision of the future becomes a new vision of faith. God stopped him in his tracks and washed away the regrets. He said to him, "Let me show you that there's more. Do not be dismayed by what you're swimming in."

When you live on the Lord's terms, there is no such thing as being eaten alive. He has you programmed to reach certain access points that end in *happily ever after*. You were built with the desires in your heart. With those desires came a magnetic plan to make them come to pass. So no matter what, you were made to impress. You have a purpose. You have a sound. You have a voice. You are a visionary. Best of all, you are an organ that works to move the larger Body of Christ.

You are made up of tissues, which serve as your goals. Your tissues are made up of cells, which function as your biological traits. Maybe you're skilled in the arts, maybe you have the gift of comfort, or maybe you're a sponge for learning new things. These are the foundation of your life, and the life of the Kingdom. Depression has not stolen your desires. It's impossible for someone to steal what God has already sealed. Depression has made you thirstier to reveal them. You are the owner of the visions imprinted on your heart. You will manifest. The hour has come for you to soak those aspirations in the river of guarantee.

Now take a second and praise Him for this eye-opener, for you've learned that faith does not rest on human wisdom, but on God's power alone. (see 1 Corinthians 2:5 NIV)

20/70: Becoming the One and Only

When I imagined the degree I had been called, I resided in a gray area for a short time. My birth was in the loading zone. I could see where Christ wanted to take me, but He needed to prep me for it first. Shutting down the world around me, including my phone, entertainment, and drawn-out lifestyle, helped me clear my schedule for a spiritual makeover. In their places, I had coffee, lunch, and dinner with God as often as I could; let me tell you, this was empowering. When you give much of your 86,400 seconds a day to the Father, you get paid for it. You cash in your wants, and He returns to you a hundred fold. That's how God runs things. Remembering this is the hard part, though.

We forget that even our deepest wants are tiny compared with how far He wants to take us. Therefore, we tend to skip out on the filling of our cups. The vision seems so close and still so far away. We devote too much energy trying to chase a thing we haven't been polished for. We skip ahead to level ten, when we've only been trained for five. You cannot jump off a cliff without bungee straps and expect to live. He's a God of order, not of destruction. He refuses to mail you in the priority batch if you haven't been processed yet.

I'd say this phase is the most critical of the three. 20/70 invites an angel to help us grow partially blind to the natural, as he flashes us into the insight of Spirit. This downgrade in acuity permits the Lord to cut off the fat and unwanted calories, while He gets us ready. What we should do in this gray area is take a knee, rest, and reset, so He can fill us with the oil needed to nurture our visions.

See it as the perfect time to write down your dreams. Create short-term goals, those that are six months or less, and high-reaching long-term goals. Write them down. Studies show that you focus on things better when they're written down. Your brain works twice as fast to store the data it collects. Make your immediate goals reasonable, because you'll be fragile after your deliverance.

Your long shots, though, need to be as ridiculous as you can make them. Outrageous ideas are always God's voice telling you to think bigger.

Once you've written down your goals, form a daily routine that will help to activate your vision. Have a morning schedule that involves chanting a brief list of affirmations. The Bible says, "Whatever is true, whatever is noble, whatever is right, whatever is pure, whatever is lovely, whatever is admirable—anything in excellence or praise—think on these things." (see Philippians 4:8) The author of this book is professing the influence of thought. What a woman thinks of herself, she becomes. What a woman speaks about herself will either unfold her purpose or melt it. Your thoughts control your identity. Therefore, dump the misery and redesign the truth.

The first five minutes of your day should be given into optimism. When you power on in the mornings, don't arise right away. In fact, set your alarm five minutes earlier than you have to be up. Use the extra time to lie in your bed for a few moments and build your mind. Start with an easy breathing exercise. Inhale for three seconds. Exhale for three. After you've sent "chill out" signals to your brain, repeat these vision-related affirmations:

1. Today, I will be led by Grace, for she will keep me in all of my ways.
2. I trust in the provision of the Spirit that I may activate the unlimited supply of riches.
3. I am a significant puzzle piece to mankind. Without my manifestation, creation is unrefined.

Copy these statements to your mirror, planner, notecards that are taped to your nightstand or dashboard of your car, or type them on your computer or phone. Refer to them throughout the day if you need a pick-me-up. When insecurities show up at work, school, or in your personal life, take a moment to cherish yourself. God has given you a vision that no one else has the rights to. You are the only one who can do you, so pocket that.

Now, let's talk about your night routine.

After a day of facing the crazy world, nights should be dedicated to restoration and fulfillment. Your actions in the evening contribute to the possibilities of tomorrow. When you're sleeping, your body is at rest, but your brain is available for premium downloads. Capitalize on this. Your routine should include journaling all of the baggage that's been sitting on your heart all day, eating the Word, reviewing and researching your goals, and securing them with a quick prayer of boldness:

"Lord, I thank You for a brand new set of lenses. I thank You that although my eyes have been led astray by the useless teachings of the Enemy, You have offered me a way out. I ask that You place a spirit of boldness in me. Secure my dreams, oh God. Produce in me a new work, and I will glorify Your name forever more. Amen."

20/200: Walking in the Calling

To trial a product means to assess its suitability or performance.[2] As an example sentence the Oxford Dictionary says, "All seeds are carefully trialed in a variety of growing conditions."

When life hits you, it knocks you over most of the time.

There is no such thing as a hair of a struggle or a mini adversity. Life is hard, no doubt. We all smell it differently, but at the end of the day, it's still called life. Because of the mud that we fall into, searching for Jesus's hand seems ludicrous. We get frustrated during the test:

"How am I supposed to have faith when it seems like there is no way out of this?"

Listen, I get it. I really do. That's the million-dollar question every believer has asked. Some have successfully walked in faith. Others have not. But the successful ones live in God's favor. The secret is that they've been trained to walk miles ahead of conflict, while looking through a glass, darkly. They have an obscure interpretation of what's real, accepting the good and ditching the horrible. In other words, becoming legally blind, or 20/200, will set you up to become rightfully bound by the Spirit. I am not implying that you will never get off track, just that you'll be put back into position with a little water and sunlight. You are a seed that has to be trialed in a variety of growing conditions to flourish.

Remember our friend Paul? Paul was legally blind. The Lord took away his sight for three days before He preached his first sermon. During those days, Paul did not eat nor drink and had to be led by nothing but a hand and a voice. He had no other option than to depend on God. Sometimes, it'll take a period of suffering for you to learn how to have faith in the blindness of things.

Take my current situation as an illustration. We're in the middle of a pandemic, I'm pregnant with our third and final Word, I'm homeschooling my eight-year old daughter, my husband is a frontline employee, and I'm scrambling to finish this book. For 11 weeks and counting, I've suffered from nausea, extreme bloat, shortness of breath, pulsatile tinnitus, heartburn, difficulty walking, migraines, swollen legs, a broken pelvis, sciatica pain, and severe muscle tears. If that's not enough, I've also been diagnosed with placenta previa, which has placed me on pelvic rest until delivery. Reading, writing, praying, and keeping the faith have been the hardest things to do. Knowing my history with stress and mental illness, I could have easily called it quits. Yet in the middle of all of this, the Lord is teaching me how to trash the bad and love on the vision. I'm crying, "Why, God? Why am I suffering the hardest in a pregnancy You told me to have? I chose to follow Your will for my life, and I feel like it's ripping me apart!"

These have been sincere conversations with my Father. He has listened, been patient, and encouraged me to stand up and walk nonetheless: "I needed these gifts in the world anyway, but you were the best and greatest person for the job. I have not led you wrong. I am with you."

Each time I hear these words in my heart, they hit me farther down than the bottom of the ocean floor. Then I begin to consider the many visions that He imparts on all people. Are we all holding on to certain gifts that we are refusing to birth? Gifts that are tethered to our personal greatness? Gifts that the world is begging us for? Are we afraid of disappointing God? Disappointing ourselves? Afraid of the embarrassment if we somehow fail? Afraid of the frustration that we might not be able to control?

If that's the case, hold back no more.

God does not fear our anger, grief, or bitterness along the walk. He welcomes it. That's what you call a true relationship. I cannot say that we will ever understand His ways, though I am sure that they are always perfect. Sufferance is faith in training. Remove the suffering, and you're powerless. Walk through it, and you're invincible. Faith gives us access to His grace, and grace activates the sauce that supersizes us on the journey. The greater the call, the greater the grace. With it, our visions are made crystal and complete. He sends us out into the wasteland and leads with His voice and the bloody prints of His hands, marking our trails with His I-AM-ness.

By faith, we build ourselves up in the density of God's love and endurance. (see Jude 1:20-21 NIV) By faith, we can do anything. We can walk on water. We can tell the wind and waves to obey us. We can heal the sick. We can raise the dead. We can reshape marriages. We can build a wealthy business. Walking in your calling means to put on your goals as if they were your skin. Exist in them. Trust in their covering. If He gave you the vision, He gave you the suit to make it happen in. The only monkey in the middle is fear. Throw him out, and all you'll have left to depend on *is* faith. This is why you must shut off your physical eye and keep the spiritual eye responsive. Fear can only live in the flesh. Deactivate the "I can't," and reactivate the "I will."

Leave doubt behind and kiss the truth. "My life is a mess, you wouldn't understand." Keep walking anyway. "My boss is trying to ruin my career." Keep walking anyway. "My husband left me for another woman." Keep walking anyway. "My children were taken from me." Keep walking anyway. "I was abused." Keep walking anyway. There are a million reasons to throw in the towel, but here's one reason not to that trumps them all: You have lived to tell the story.

That said, He's not finished with you. Push through the brokenness. For it is only in your force that you will figure out what's on the other side. I promise you that whatever He has is beyond anything you could think or ask. Take a chance on yourself. Hitting rock bottom is how you rebuild a structure. What can stop you now? *Who* can stop you now?

The call is worth it.

The walk is worth it.

The tears are worth it.

You are worth it.

Keep going, Sis. You got this.

THE *Access*

Father grants you the universal keycard. He then gives you permission to go **HAM**: You have access to His **H**eart, His **A**uthority, and His **M**ind.

Part One: Be Intentional with His Ventricles

The human heart is split into four chambers. Those chambers are two atria and two ventricles. Both atria receive blood and pumps it to the ventricles. The right ventricle sends deoxygenated blood to the lungs to be purified and packed with oxygen. The left ventricle pumps the newly oxygenated blood to the aorta to be distributed to the rest of the body. I love this process. Every part of the heart knows its job, and they work together to complete a task that receives the same results over, and over, and over again. More than 100,000 times per day, blood is pumped throughout the body. They never get tired of working as a team because there are no small parts. If one chamber becomes damaged, stiff, or weak, the rest of the heart will thicken and expand to compensate.

Assume the human heart functions the same as the heart of God. The heart of God is the Son of God, and the Son is the Life of the world. Inasmuch as He voluntarily gave Himself up for us, we have been fastened to a legally binding contract, one that states, "No one can come to the Father except through the Son." (see John 14:6) After the Fall, God made a pact with mankind. He agreed to forgive all of our sins from the past, present, and future succeeding the heroic acts of a living Sacrifice. Once the Lord's spirit was emancipated, the Father's heart *for* man became the Heart *of* man, "I am persuaded that neither death, nor life, nor angels, nor principalities, nor powers, nor things present, nor things to come, nor height, nor depth, nor any other creature, shall be able to separate us from the love of God, *which is in* Christ Jesus our Lord." (Romans 8:38-39)

The Son was given a special seat, smack dab in the center of His Activated Body. He got us pumping again! This time, indefinitely. He healed the diastasis—the manual separation between the people and Elohim. He alleviated the burden by becoming the burden, our iniquity and pain. This granted us access to the largest availability of God. Christ wasn't just another prophet. He was the New Order. A cardiac DJ. The heart of the Body moves by the tempo of His record, making Him a Master at the ones and twos. The Father surrendered it all to Him because He trusted His Son with the cries of His people.

The issues that exist today are managed by that same honor and love. If you could peek inside the Father's heart, you'd see the Son, and if you look inside the Son's heart, you'd see yourself. The world lives in Him, Who lives in Him. As certified by the Cross.

Let's revisit the deal I was referring to earlier.

Our servanthood came with a contract; as with many legally binding contracts, it has six key elements. I have to mention though, this one is fairly unique. This contract displays God's affection toward humanity:

1. **The offer: One party makes a proposition.** Jesus paid for your room in Heaven and offered you to be His roommate.

2. **The acceptance: The other party accepts the offer laid on the table.** He laid down His life for you. Are you willing to pick it up and put it to good use in your heart?

3. **Consideration: Each party must make a promise**

or present an act. Keep in mind that His offering, which was both a promise and an act, encourages you to present yourself as a holy and acceptable sacrifice for Him.

4. **Mutuality of obligation: Both parties must be able to perform their obligations.** God patiently holds up His side of the bargain. Your dedication to Him is the single transaction needed on your part.

5. **Competency and capacity: Both parties must understand that they've entered into a contract.** Jesus's word is His bond. Can you secure yours, likewise? Here's a hint: The only thing He needs from you is loyalty.

6. **The written statement: This is the statement that seals the deal.** 66 books of Holy Scripture can attest to this divine law. *And just in case you were wondering, no, this contract never expires. Glory be to God!*

After signing the contract, Jesus gives you access to the intentions of His heart. He uses you the way His other Half used Him—to cover the bills. You are chosen to help with the world's pain.

Untrained mindsets

Emotional despair

Thorns in flesh

Oppression

A desire for more

Mayhem

Despite what some believe, grief signals aren't trashy news to the Lord. He doesn't flip the channel on our pain. When the people call, He answers. When we need Him, He delivers. Our blood cries out to God from the ground like Abel's did when he was murdered. With more than 4.54 billion years under His belt, He has an amazing system in place for the earth's tears. We are that system, His children. By equipping the chosen generation, His solution for hardship is sent through four chambers before it can be fulfilled. This flow develops a crisp heart in the royal Body.

I am sure you've learned by now that nothing about the Father is done out of order. He coaches us in all things, including how to love.

Take a closer look at how a cry out to God is answered through the ones He has called:

The First Chamber: Agape

- In humans, the right atrium receives deoxygenated blood and sends it to the right ventricle via the tricuspid valve. This valve is a triple-door access for optimal retrieval.
- In the Body of Christ, the right atrium hears the cries from around the globe and accepts them with the highest form of love, agape. This is a pure, unselfish, intentional, sacrificial kind of love that is concerned about the good of all people. The Trinity is a triple-door access of agape. God *is* Love. He takes care of us with the same love He created us with. That's all it took to design us; that's all it takes to restore us. Love tears down strongholds and mends the impossible. We are taught to

resolve every affair in love, (see Galatians 5:13-14) because it covers a multitude of sin.

The Second Chamber: Foundation

- In humans, the right ventricle receives blood from the right atrium and sends it to the lungs to be filled with oxygen.

- In the Body of Christ, this is our first pumping brief. We accept the heart of God and use it to build a foundation in our own hearts. The gifts planted in us are like oxygen. They're put there to serve others. But our hearts must be in it before we can help a soul. To do this, we have to step back and ask ourselves, "Is my heart built on purity, or am I holding on to some things that could hinder my service in Kingdom?"

  Father desires for us to honor one another above ourselves. Because most of us don't do that naturally, He takes our love to be cleansed and fabricated on a rock. That rock acts as the lungs. It is the site of transfer, where sinful nature is exchanged for a "rock and a hard place." Originally, this saying was written to explain a series of possibilities that all end in difficulty. In this context, however, I am talking about the great wall of God. It's a place where no matter how you use it, the love that you spread will be firm and functional because it was built by Jesus. This chamber shreds any division between you and the Messiah, you and the people, or you and yourself. It replaces selfishness with selflessness.

The Third Chamber: Fire

- In a human heart, the left atrium grabs the new blood from the lungs and delivers it to the left ventricle.

- In the Lord's Body, our foundation is partnered with a relentless torch. This is the stuff that gets us fired up for God, ready to do His work. I witnessed this chamber in prayer one day. It was an early Saturday morning, and I was under loads of mental pressure. I was desperate for a power surge. I asked Holy Spirit to let me know that He was listening. I wanted some sort of a sign. As my heart lifted toward Heaven and my hands opened in the symbol of acceptance, He gave me a vision. I began to watch a flame elevate from the palms of my hands, which were at my waist, and rise to my eyes. I was on fire! I remember thinking, *Not only are You listening, but You're showing me how critical it is to persevere.*

  When God uses us, He gets us fired up. Zeal is important to Him. Without zeal, we drown in our own sweat. This is why God puts a fire to your bum, to get you up and out. You see, the human heart has to be put under pressure, blood pressure, in order for the blood to move throughout the body. If the blood doesn't move fast enough, your organs will shut down. We have to understand that God will put us under pressure to get things done for Him. The pressure shouldn't produce a panic, though. It should produce a flame.

The Fourth Chamber: Replenish

- In humans, this is the last chamber. The left ventricle pumps the oxygenated blood to the aorta and out to the rest of the body.

- In the House, this is our final pumping session. Like a breastfeeding mother pumps out milk for her baby, we are to squeeze out the milk of God and moisturize the land on which we stand. It is a call to replenish the earth. To replenish means to fill again. This is what preserves His heartbeat. This is how the Body stays active. This is what keeps the people clenched to the care packages from Heaven. The blessings come from God, they stream through the gifts of the chosen, and finally, they're gushed out to fulfill a cry. We are to accept the world's pain with love, build a strong foundation, light our gifts on fire, and reload mankind through the multi-door outlets.

Up until now, we've been educated on the character of love and how we play a huge part in rebuilding the Body. But you may be asking yourself, *How can I be intentional with His ventricles? What is my role in all of this? Am I only to use His intentions to save the world and not myself?*

Allow me to answer the last question before I touch on the first two. God initially works to strengthen you (recall the second chamber, *the foundation*). Your heart and mind are stepping stones for maturation. If you're not strengthened, how can He use you to edify others? He satiates you before you can feed them. Simple enough, right? As for the previous inquiries, being intentional involves three strides:

1. **First and foremost, you have to know what hurts God's heart and be mindful that He is still in**

control. In addition to the cries I called out before, unbelief in Him or yourself is a major contributor to His pain. He needs you to believe. That's why He says to enter His gates like a child: because children have faith. They dream of the impossible. Adults are used to their ways and unwilling to change. So backtrack the age of your compassion for Him. Go back to the time when you were trusting, expectant, and loving. Bring out that childlike faith again. This will show you God's heart and stop you from questioning whether or not He can overrule an issue.

2. **Secondly, whatever hurts Him should hurt you**. If it doesn't, step number three will seem impractical.

3. **Lastly, find creative ways to heal creation**. This is where the release of your ministry steps in. Most people see ministry as a tie to the church, but that's not accurate. The word "ministry" literally means the work of God, not the work of God in a church building. In view of this, ministry is everywhere. Architecture is a ministry; science is a ministry; medicine is a ministry; baking is a ministry; photography is a ministry. Teaching, painting, parenting, friendship, poetry, and styling hair are all ministries. Heck, even working at McDonald's is doing God's work.

   One extraordinary thing that each of those jobs, careers, and callings have in common is people. Consider the Lord's visionary statement: "My command is this: Love each other as I have loved you." (John 15:12) He uses people to creatively love on people.

Loving one another is the solution to saving one another. It's the solution to an abundant life. When you start to look at the work of God as being of service to others, showing kindness throughout, you'll be able to usher in the fragrance of the Lord in anything you do, anything you say, and anywhere you go. A hug may cure PTSD. A complement could reverse depression. A plain ol' smile could make a difference.

I remember getting my blood drawn at a prenatal appointment when I met a beautiful soul of a woman. She was the phlebotomy tech. As my blood rushed into the tube, she looked at me and said, "You are glowing! Is this your first baby?"

I responded, "Aw, thank you. But no, this is my third child."

She said, "I would have never thought!"

I smiled and replied, "Oh, that's just the glory of God."

With a surprised look on her face, she said, "Well, amen to that, sweetheart! I love it!"

Upon completing the blood draw, my comment was brought up once more, "Wow, thank you for what you said earlier. You have truly blessed me today."

Her reply stunned me. All I did was speak from the sincerity of my heart, nothing more. But she saw it as a blessing. Who knows, she could have been losing her faith that day, and I reminded her of God's love.

I wasn't hunting to bless anyone. I wasn't trying to preach or teach. I just happened to be in the right place at the right time, and the Father used my words as a creative way to heal creation. How wonderful is that? To pronounce His love into simple words and deeds in the middle of our day, we can express the heart of God without even trying.

There's a purity in your light, one that follows you wherever you go, and that light is used to save His people.

Spend the remainder of your life on agape currency—learning to love in actions and in truth day by day (1 John 3:18 NIV)—because you never know who needs it.

Part Two: Stand in Command

To stand in command means to give an authoritative order; to dominate from a superior height or elevated place.[3]

There's an old story of a man whose hometown didn't accept him. This man had multitudes being healed from the cloth on his back. He raised the bar of intelligence as we know it. He put a three-day tab on his death. He had demons begging him not to crush them. This man's name is Jesus. He was given unanimous authority before time, in time, and past time. He is the Pioneer of the word *command*, teaching us to be resilient even when our minds have come against us, even as we're being nailed to a cross.

Women, who are seen as the weak gender, should staple

God's authority to their foreheads when doubting their impact. We have always gotten the short end of the stick. No matter how many times it has been broken in half, we are given the undersized end.

Get a load of corporate America. Men perform identical roles as females, but they're often paid a whopping 10 to 20, and in some cases, 50 percent higher than women. For what? Because of the differences in parts? How biased is that! After working to land your dream job, you get stiffed on the perks next to some guy.

And women generally face discrimination across the board, not just in the workplace.

We are targeted for sexual offense, domestic violence, unjust marriages, gender partialities in the immigration system, and zero entitlement to our bodies. Hundreds of millions of women from Africa and the Middle East are mutilated as young girls because people want to dismiss their sexual rights. This degrading and inhumane practice has caused these poor children hemorrhaging, problems urinating, infections, childbirth complications, shock, and even death. To what end? Because they shouldn't be able to explore something biologically granted to them by God? While men from these same countries are walking around fully equipped and freely doing however they please. It's awful what women have put up with for so long. No wonder feminism was born. These breaches in gender equality have always been around, essentially longer than the days of racial slavery.

I recall a Samaritan woman from the Bible who was scorned for having five husbands and fornicating with a sixth man. This lady would have to go out in the heat to fetch water just to avoid humiliation by her neighbors. I can only imagine the self-doubt that met her day and night, pondering on her actions and being crammed with guilt. She was privately coping through depression. But all of that changed when she received a visit from Christ one afternoon. He did away with the separation between Jews and Samaritans, and He ended the gender gap as well. He told her, and I'm paraphrasing here, "You don't have to live inferior to anyone. Let Me show you the importance of female empowerment. I can offer you a drink from a living well, and in this, you'll be activated for life."

She left that chat with dignity. Her personal visitation from God went on to inspire those in her circle to find the Source of endless water. They thought, *If this woman can face us in her shame, surely, she'd been with the Savior*. He used the weak to shame the strong.

There's something missing from that story, though. Where were the five men, and why weren't they scorned? I'm sure they'd been married a few times. Hey, they could have cheated on the woman, which caused her several marriages. See, questions like these baffle me. Rituals were coerced on the gentle sex, even down to killing them for adultery. Yet the men involved were given a pat on the butt and told to keep up the good work. Sounds like sexism to me. Luckily, we can learn from women over the course of history who have shown us that authority *does* exist in the female. Women who have inspired us to fight for what we deserve. Our opinions, our rights, our voices do matter.

In 1776, Abigail Adams wrote a letter to her husband

to balance the power between genders. She urged John and the Continental Congress to remember the ladies or face the repercussions of a rebellion. She penned, "We will not hold ourselves bound by any laws in which we have no voice or representation." Her bravery, added with a long list of daring women after, was the reason for the Nineteenth Amendment 144 years later. This is the amendment that gave women the right to vote. Abigail spoke up without fear, and this empowered the generations to come:

- Florence Nightingale, a nurse who defied the odds, completely reformed healthcare in the Crimean War. She chose to care for soldiers in a filthy hospital with horrible living arrangements. Her grit initiated major respect from male doctors, and she was soon named a hero. Cheers to Florence for opening up the door for nurses to stand in command.

- Rosa Parks, a black seamstress, remained positioned in her seat after being verbally forced to move. Her refusal to stand up for a white man was a symbol of her standing in authority for her rights. Rosa's tenacity ended segregation on the city bus system and began the civil rights movement thereafter. She's a beloved activist who is still spoken of to this day, because she has taught us that even in your silence you can be heard.

- Marie Curie, a Polish scientist who co-discovered elements of radioactivity, was the first woman to win a

Nobel Prize. In fact, she won two. The first was with her husband, and the second was on her own. We can thank her for x-rays and treatments in the medical field. Her research saves millions of lives every day.

I can make this list go on forever, but I think you get the point. The female is unstoppable. She is authoritative. She is resilient. She is...the Man. Emphasis on that capital "M." Christ has shared His commanding fist with you. You can rule as He does. Darkness must obey *you*. Depression has to yield to *you*. Standing against your disorder should not be intimidating; it should be enabling, because the woman reading this can do whatever, and I mean whatever, she wills to do in life.

There's a statement Holy Spirit placed in my heart regarding my command on earth, one that has really stuck with me to this day. After my deliverance, I began sensing the presence of my guardian angel on the left of me. Curious as to why he preferred that side, I asked the Lord for answers, "God, why do I always feel an angelic presence on my left?"

His response was direct, "Because you're my right-hand man."

It warmed my spirit when I thought about how true this was. People are the embodiment of the Creator. He never said His angels mirrored His reflection. He said we do. "He makes His angels spirits, and His servants flames of fire." (Hebrews 1:7 NIV) They're beautifully made by God as well, but they are purely ministering spirits sent to serve those who will inherit salvation." (Hebrews

1:14 NIV) Out of everything the Architect has built, His sons and daughters have been given the highest place as sovereign rulers over the four corners of the globe.

So when you start feeling mediocre, remember that you are God's right-hand. Marry that authority. Become intimate with it. When you snap your fingers, you should view the whole world as a platform that is expecting to hear from the Man in you. You have the power to claim what's yours. Do not go around thinking you don't deserve something just because another person seems better for it, nor because you think God favors them. You have every tool needed to prosper. Never underrate yourself. What the Lord gives you is yours for good. Ascribe to that. Know who's operating in you. Know who's guarding your spine.

I dare you to wake up today and see yourself above all else. I dare you to command your atmosphere. I dare you to go out and start proclaiming the words:

"I'm the Man! I refuse to be whipped into the shape of inferiority. I am the outsider who's getting ready to change the inside."

Part Three: Retain His Brain

There are more than 80 billion neurons in the human brain.[4] This collection of cells can analyze the wheel of color that meets the eye, your threshold of pain, the moment you fall in love, the second you get hungry, and the minute you're stricken by the cold. Your reality is reported by a mass number of building blocks. With all of those cells, it's a miracle our brains don't explode. One would think, right? The brain is designed to hold at least 2,500,000 gigabytes of storage. Some say it's enough space to hold the entire internet! Clearly, the sky is the limit for this organ.

A healthy person is blessed with the beauty of their brain. A depressed person, on the other hand, is trying to reach the bare minimum. When someone is severely depressed, their brains aren't reaching the sky. They aren't even getting up off of the ground. Their senses have gone numb. Their memory is nonexistent. Their storage is the size of a breadcrumb. Instead of becoming a fully functional unit of intelligence, their brain has become like mush: useful for absolutely nothing. Being freed from this disease is great. But know that you've been deficient for some time now. Depression has muddled your nerves. It has degenerated everything in your skull. You've become dry, empty, lost, dull. New connections and pathways must be formed. We need to reforest your roots. We have to find new concepts to strengthen your thoughts.

When I fathomed the access I had to God's mind, I began tapping into it. I used His brainpower as motivation to enhance my own. If He's brilliant, then I can access that. If the human brain has been mastered, how far more incredible is the Master's brain that designed it? (see Colossians 2:3) Hugh Ross, our physicist friend from chapter five, has studied the Lord to be ten trillion, trillion, trillion, trillion, trillion, trillion, trillion, trillion times more ingenious and knowledgeable than the smartest human being.

Although I trust in the basis of Ross's research, and the numbers certainly amaze me, I have a hunch that it's on a surface level. I assume the Father is so intelligent that no one is able to calculate it without threatening their life. I say this because God tells Moses in the book of Exodus that no man can see His face and live. (Exodus 33:20) He's only talking about *seeing* His face here. If we're unable to picture the outside of the Creator's head without dying, what makes anyone think they'd be able to compute the networks on the inside?

Nevertheless, the takeaway is this: The Lord is smarter than we know, and we can have some of that. We should know His thoughts, something that develops with reading and praying, and we should take advantage of the visionary box He's given us. We ought to use the good of human fitness, instead of the laziness that we often fall into the trap of. (see 3 John 1:11) The accepted style of using our brains is to spend hours on social media, watching television, and thinking about vanity all day long, "What's a good show on Netflix to binge?" "Did you see this post, girl?" "I need to make sure I pick up a new set of lashes today."

This kind of talk is normal. This kind of sense is common. Yet customs aren't always good to follow. I guarantee you that they are the number one reason for the global decline in IQ over recent years. All of humanity has some sort of a mental decline this day and age.

A lack of self-control

Problems staying focused

Subpar retention, you name it

With so much information readily accessible at our fingertips, we basically have to force-feed our brains the exact opposite of what it's receiving from society's kitchen. We have to challenge the norm. Let me share with you a few things that gave my brain the food it needed to bounce back and liven up:

† **Lubricate your thoughts.** If you wish to give your crown the best diamonds that the world provides, change the game up. Have a goal at the top of your bucket list that says, "I'm going to commit myself to gaining A1 intelligence. If God has a gorgeous brain, then so is the one He placed in me." Use Him as your incentive to discover as much as you can before leaving earth. Instead of waking up and saying good morning to the notifications on your phone, greet brainpower. Open up Spotify and listen to educational podcasts. If those don't interest you, type in "motivational speeches" or "brain hacks" on YouTube and bask in those. Allow these outlets to seep into your mind as you're taking a shower, brushing your teeth, or making breakfast. They'll pump you up the same as a cup of coffee and jumpstart your day.

   In addition to this, create a habit of reading during your leisure time. Search for books that cover topics related to mental stamina and go ham. Learn from them. Place the information wherever it fits in your life-bubble. Your brain must be exercised to build new connections, just as you would work out your abdomen to build a new six-pack.

† **Be present in the moment.** Because memory and focus are lessened by depression, conversations and tasks can be

dreadful. When depressed, your natural tendency is to dodge people and responsibilities that demand your energy. But what I've learned from doing this is that I would never get better if I didn't practice at becoming human again. Sure, it sounds odd to train in the artistry of personhood. But it is vital for your healing.

Try hugging every moment with your fullest attention. Don't run from small talk with a stranger, give it your all by using the three R's: relax your body from mind to soul, receive emotional cues from the other person (making it your duty to really hear and feel what they're saying to you), and respond. During the chat, do not feel the need to impress. Nor should you bash your responses with a hammer. Just be present. Take everything in and go with the wave. Also, keep in mind that Holy Spirit can jump in and speak for you if you ever need Him to. Just pray about it.

When it comes to checking off your daily goals, obey the same rule as above. Dive into the moment. Give every task its own special care. If you're cleaning, play some music and enjoy that time to love on your home. If you're working, silence any distractions. If you're studying, tie yourself to the material. If you give everything your undivided attention, it'll be a lot easier to pull from your memory blog and speed up your focus.

✝ **Dissect and redirect your physical.** Get your blood tested. Find out if there are any imbalances that you *can* change right away. For example, I'm anemic, so taking iron supplements helps with that. Whenever I'm not taking them, I sense it. I lack energy and can't find my center. Know your body and give it what it needs to run a marathon. I also suggest eating a wholesome diet. Stock up on fruits, veggies, protein, whole grains and omega-3 fatty acids, and drink a ton of water.

Many people hate to admit this, but if you feed the brain crappy food all the time, you'll see crappy results come out of it. Physical health is brain wealth.

ACT
on this!

I invite you on a 33-day self-love challenge. The number 33 is a numerical code for the word "amen." If you were to assign a number to each letter of the alphabet in order from 1 to 26, A would be the number 1, M would be 13, E would be 5, and N would be 14. Altogether that equals 33. Amen can be defined as "Thy will be done." God's will is for you to truly love yourself the way He loves you. Thus, for 33 days, I want to challenge you to spin a daily "amen." Look into the mirror completely naked and hug or touch the areas of your body that you are self-conscious about. Show yourself love by repeating this mantra three times in a row: "Through the love of God, I have been made perfect and complete. Every part of my body is a symbol of breathtaking beauty and strength. I am in love with me." By the end of the challenge, journal your thoughts about it. Has your confidence improved? And remember to give yourself grace during this, as the slightest bit of change is a win for you.

"

YOU ARE NO LONGER ACTING OUT YOUR OWN IMAGE. YOU HAVE BEEN SELECTED TO PLAY THE ROLE OF GOD.

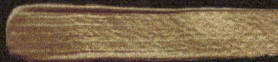

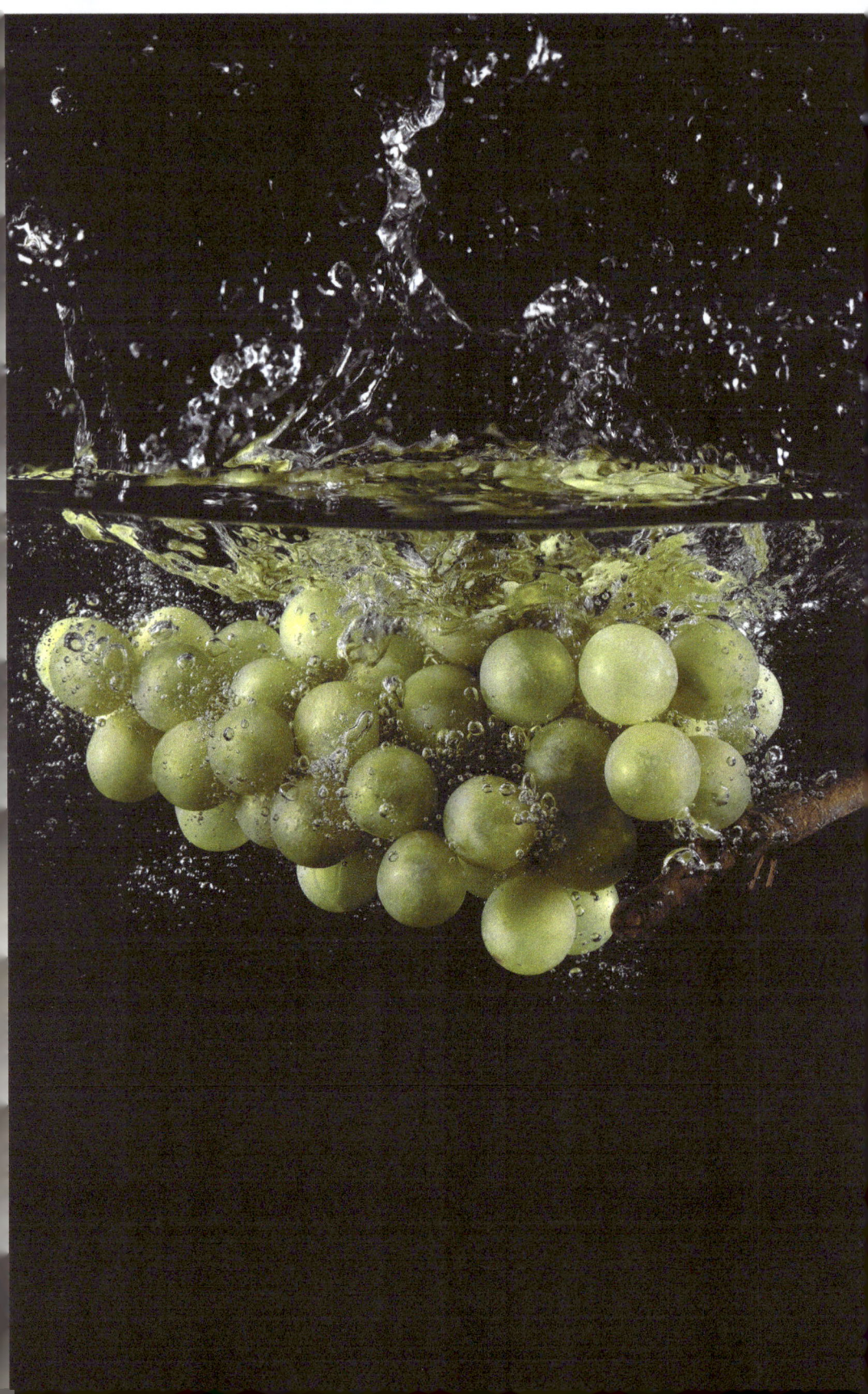

CHAPTER EIGHT

THE LAST TRIMESTER

Fruits of the Spirit

This is really happening. It's month nine, and the mother's body is getting ready to welcome her new creation. She's apprehensive, enthusiastic, and maybe a little restless. She's finally gotten the chance to feel the "quickening"—the baby's kicks—and the two of them are closer than ever. Mommy and baby have become one. When Mommy eats, baby eats. When Mommy breathes, baby breathes. When Mommy's heart beats, baby's follows. They are on one accord. She's learned about her child, and he has seen the innermost parts of her. Their steps have been ordered in purpose, together. They share the same blood, the same water, the same body.

Through God's nine-month-long presence in your womb, you've beaten the odds. You've even felt the quickening, those rivers of life that flood your belly. As you've eaten the Pages, the Spirit in you has been fed. As your heart has pounded, so has His. As you've inhaled truth, He's exhaled wisdom through you. You are now a firstfruit, for *"Every good and perfect gift is from above, coming down from the Father of the heavenly lights, who does not change like shifting shadows. He chose to give us birth through the word of truth, that we might be a kind of firstfruits of all He created."* (James 1:17-18)

This chapter is the last training session before labor. It's time for a richer devotion and expression of Jesus. The previous phases educated you on His virtues and your place in Kingdom. This phase tacks on bodybuilding—a complete ensemble of Holy Spirit.

THE Trademark

A **trademark** is a symbol or word legally registered by use as representing a company or a product. We are the trademark of the Melchizedek Priest, the representation of the King. (see Hebrews 6:17-20 NIV) As the symbol of His three-part brand, we have to trade our mark for His. You are to live in the Word-ness of things versus the you-ness of things. This trade is done in three ways: learning to follow Christ, maintaining His composure during the good fight, and relentlessly sharing the Gospel.

Part 1: Led by Liquid Red

Blood is a four-part substance. It is made up of plasma, red blood cells, white blood cells, and platelets. The functions of this mix include transporting, clotting, warding, filtering, and regulating body temperature.

Blood intrigues me, mainly because it perfectly resembles the blood of Christ. The red liquid that was shed for you on Calvary provides a coverage as well. It nourishes you, seals you, kills off pathogens, cleanses you, and steadies you under Heaven. You become the emblem of God, copyrighted and distributed for greater works. Advocating for this Company should not be seen as imprisonment. Rather, view it as an opportunity, a chance to be led by liquid red.

When you slip on the dress of the Spirit, you model that dress in front of people who are desperately hunting for a new look. You are a fresh beacon of hope for them. They watch you, they want to become you, and they'll spend the rest of their lives getting to know the God in you. Deep down, we all want to be mentally sound, kind, patient, and self-controlled. We just never know where to start. We don't even believe that's possible for one who was born into sin. I imagine that every person has faced the universal query a few times: "How can I become a better person?"

Famished to plug in that void, we spend time reading articles and watching videos that claim to tutor us on character building, the kind that are titled, *Ten Life Skills to Improve your Personality*. Here's my concern with these channels though: If these people aren't teaching from the roles of the Spirit, you are technically just snacking on almonds. They're offering you sampled food from Publix and calling it fulfillment. But how could anyone maintain enough energy from an appetizer? It's unreasonable, wouldn't you agree? Stop expecting those tiny pieces of protein to match your dietary guidelines for the day. Practice activating a real seed of growth and development. Lunch on the fruit basket of oil.

This is where the word "act" really comes in to play. Think of this step as the final exam taken in your senior year of high school, the ACT. Get serious about it. Study for it. Live for it. Shift the focus from acting out your own imperfect image, to betrothing the perfect image of God.

So, how do we undertake His character exactly? Don't make this too complicated. The only way to become someone else is to duplicate their mannerisms. Lucky for us, the Lord has already outlined His fruit in Scripture:

1. Show love. Love is a blend of all nine fruits. Love is patient, love is kind; it does not envy or boast; it is not full of pride; it does not dishonor others; it is not self-seeking; it is not easily angered; it keeps no record of wrongs; it does not delight in evil but rejoices in truth. Love always protects, trusts, hopes, and perseveres. (see 1 Corinthians 13:4-8 NIV)

- You show love by setting aside every mode of temperament, judgment, or ideas you've been accustomed to over the years and exchanging them for this one idea: the person in front of you *is* God. Treat people with the same respect you'd give if you were staring God in the face. The Bible says, "...I was hungry and you gave Me food; I was thirsty and you gave Me drink; I was a stranger and you took Me in; I was naked and you clothed Me; I was sick and you visited Me; I was in prison and you came to Me. Then the righteous will answer Him, saying, 'Lord, when did we see You a stranger and take You in, or naked and clothe You? Or when did we see you sick, or in prison, and come to You?' And the King will answer and say to them, 'Assuredly, I say to you, inasmuch as you did it to one of the least of these My brethren, you did it to Me.'" (Matthew 25:35-40)

How you treat people is how you treat Christ. Would you call Him out of His name, refuse to offer Him your forgiveness, or turn away your shoulder when He needs it to cry on? No ma'am, you would not. Likewise, you should use that same love-power on others. Don't pay so much attention to what a person does to you. Give attention to the love you have for the Person who made them. See Him when you see them.

Now this is, in my opinion, the toughest mission to accomplish, and it takes loads of bravery to become successful at. People know how to hit emotional buttons that you never thought possible. They can summon the devil out of you and hide the pretty fragments under a rock somewhere. Nevertheless, love will be one of the most rewarding seeds of character development if you choose to plant it. Trust my word on this. I've lived with and without the use of vegetation, and to this day, I still find places in the garden of my heart to sow these love-gems.

I used to get easily offended by actions and statements fired at me. It didn't matter if they were coming from strangers, family members, or close friends. Everyone was the enemy. But the Lord has shared with me that the secret to maintaining strong relationships with anyone is to view others as Himself, finding something to love about them in those hot seats of rage, instead of occupying that time in disgust. You have to see the beauty of the Lord inside of someone's ugliness because people fall short, yet Christ is unblemished.

Practicing this has repositioned me. I'm less exhausted when I have forgiven on the spot than I am when I'm drowning in my feelings for the next couple of weeks. Or months. Or years for that matter. I'm not perfect, and God still loves me. They're not perfect either. The least I could do is love the God in them. If this seems too hard for you, remember who wore it best.

Our Savior prayed earnestly for those who were killing Him *while* it was taking place. "Father, forgive them, for they know not what they do." (Luke 23:34) He loved us so that, in order to lay down the ground rules for an eternal life, He left His Father to cleave to His Wife: us, the Body of Christ. He's the epitome of what it means to sacrifice a temporary feeling for an exemplary outcome. He's shown that when you plant love-gems, you'll reap emotional, spiritual, and relational abundance.

2. Discover joy. Joy is **J**esus **o**ver **Y**earning—accept the He that lives in you, and deny the tendency to long for more.

- We have been taught that breathing is involuntary. Giving credit to the medulla and spinal cord, our respiratory pattern is seen as an automated effort. Inhale, exhale, repeat. Sadly, this action is abused by many. We're either dying for the next big thing to knock our socks off, or we're wasting fuel on disappointment that keep us held at gunpoint on the couch, losing all hope in what tomorrow may bring. The flesh never delights in today. She never floats in the present. She's too busy running circles around the pit of ingratitude. What a fruitless life this produces! What a death label this makes.

  We're not following biblical advice when we choose tommorow's worries over today's joy. God teaches us to keep our hearts stayed upon Him when everything feels broken. Happiness is considered mental therapy. His Word says that a joyful heart is good medicine, but a crushed spirit dries up the bones." (see Proverbs 17:22 NIV) Yes, it is written that we will face troubles, but it is also written that joy comes in the morning. So, let tomorrow worry about itself, and search for happiness now.

Joy isn't far from the tears you've cried day and night. You cannot see it yet, but He's carrying your strength in His palm. He has your prosperity under a lock and key. He will restore to you the years that the swarming locust has eaten, the crawling locust, the consuming locust, and the chewing locust; you shall eat plenty and be satisfied. (see Joel 2:25) Rejoice now, in the middle of all the chaos, because tomorrow is not promised. The next hour isn't promised. Your next minute isn't promised. Nor can you rewind the clock. When time gets away, you can't call it back. There's no such thing as recycled seconds. Once they leave, they're gone for good.

Don't renege on your now moments. Study your blessings each day. Foster a habit to brew a couple of "thank yous" on the regular. Look around you. What do you see? What do you have? Who's in your circle? Is there at least one thing you can be thankful for? If nothing comes to mind, place a hand on your heart and feel it tap you. Let this be a reason to tell God thank you.

Our schoolbooks dishonor the power of the Lord by teaching us that breathing is involuntary. Dare I reveal the truth? Your next breath is not automated, it's pre-calculated. God is the stick shift behind every *inhale, exhale*. He's set the action of your lungs to the degree of which He'll use you. Therefore, take every breath as an opportunity of praise, because each time you breathe, that's 960 times per hour, 23,040 times per day, and 8,409,600 times a year that God personally added another second to your life, just to show how much you're worth to Him.

3. Find peace. Peace is the stunt double that replaces your understanding.

- According to theologians, "fear not" is the most repeated command in the Bible. 365 verses call us to be fearless. I don't believe it is a coincidence that there are also 365 days in a year. He wanted us to lift this message on a daily basis as an attempt to keep our peace. In a world, where everyone is suffering from anxieties of the unknown, especially in a pandemic, it's challenging to stay calm under pressure. The body's natural reaction is to drive itself mad, drive you to fear the worst. That's the keyword, though. You. *You* are the one driving yourself mad. But don't you know that you are your own peace pilot? You have total control over your reactions.

Life is like a science experiment. In an experiment, you maneuver the independent variable and weigh the outcome with the dependent variable. Crises are independent and always evolving. How you respond to a crisis should be the dependent variable, your remote control so to speak. Because you cannot depend on the game of life to remain stable, override it with the pause button on the remote. Keep your peace still. It's not the predicament that kills a person, it's how they respond to it.

Take the windstorm in the Bible for example. Jesus and His crew were crossing over the sea on a boat, when a violent storm arose. The storm was so fierce that the waves began to beat into the boat and cause it to start filling up. Jesus was asleep on a pillow as if nothing was happening. He was probably snoring and having a pretty good dream as well because He was totally unbothered. The disciples, on the other hand, were so fearful that they believed they were close to death, crying "Teacher, do You not care that we are perishing?" (Mark 4:38) Jesus awakened and took control, "Peace, be still!"

Suddenly, the waves stopped, and the wind calmed down. Then He continued, "Why are you so fearful? How is it that you have no faith?" The disciples looked at Him, looked at what He'd just done, and then turned to each other and shouted, "Who can this be, that even the wind and the sea obey Him!" (Mark 4:39-41)

Every single man on the boat was in the middle of the same storm that night, so what was the difference between the Lord's response and theirs? He was the only one who took advantage of peace. He made the storm fear Him, as opposed to Him panicking over it. He didn't care about the fuss it was making because He knew how to grab the wheel. In fact, He went to sleep on it!

That's the lesson here. Pretend that your brain is a remote that controls your frame of mind. A remote usually has the options to mute the TV, play, pause, rewind, and fast forward. With the arrows and menu buttons, it also has the option to set a sleep timer. Let the anxieties you face become the TV, and use your remote to put them to sleep. Make the attacks be afraid of you. Cause the Enemy to have to upgrade his mouse traps. Don't make it easy for him. Go to sleep on him! Have faith that against all odds, God always wins over fear.

The Word testifies that if we believe that Jesus died and rose for us, God will bring with Him those who sleep in Jesus. (see 1 Thessalonians 4:14) He gives the peace that guards the heart and mind. "Fear not, for I am with you. Be not dismayed, for I am your God. I will strengthen you. I will uphold you with My righteous right hand." (Isaiah 41:10) If *He's* upholding us, the Engineer Himself, this alone should give you a reason to sleep it off.

4. Be patient. Patience is having the capacity to tolerate delay, trouble, or suffering without getting angry or upset.

- Here it is, the first month of the year 2021, and I gave birth to my third child in October of last year. Due to the ripping of my muscles and breaking of my bones during the pregnancy, he had room to grow as big as he wanted. Jace's birth weight was nine pounds and fourteen ounces. Yes, girl, I pushed out nearly a ten-pound baby! I often joke with others and say he came out with a driver's license and headed to college. Not only was the postpartum recovery the hardest out of all my children, but Jace hated diaper changes, being in the swing, taking baths, sitting in his carseat, and sleeping by himself, not to mention his major tummy issues. For the first few weeks, he wanted Mommy. Nothing or no one else would suffice. He'd scream at the top of his lungs if you'd try and fight him on that. Exhausted from never having a minute to breathe, or rest, or even finish writing my book that I'd been eager to complete, I gave God the side eye.

  "Do You even care what I'm going through, Lord?"

  Obviously, I was asking the wrong question

because He didn't respond. A few weeks passed, and I had the courage to do what most believers don't. I decided to change the question. Instead of asking Him why this was happening to me, I asked what He was trying to teach me.

The Spirit said, "Patience."

Being the human that I am and always thinking I know so much, I said to Him: "But God I'm already..."

Before I could even finish the sentence, He stopped me: "If you were, I wouldn't have to teach it to you, now would I?"

He was right. As always. I hadn't been patient. Annoyed is what I was. Annoyed because Jace was unplanned and seemed to delay my book being released. Annoyed because I was in pain, couldn't fit into my wardrobe, and felt that all of my wants and needs were on pause. The truth is, I failed at being patient. I lacked the capacity to tolerate delay, trouble, or suffering without getting angry or upset. Our talk helped me change my attitude that night. From that day forward, I chose to look ahead. *This too shall pass* has been the sermon that I've preached to myself since then, and guess what? Things have gotten better.

Jace, at three months old, now sleeps 9 to 12 hours per night in his own bed, he laughs during diaper changes and baths, and he's building a new relationship with his carseat. You can't tell me my God isn't good! Allow my story to encourage you. The Father doesn't magically save you from affliction. He's fully capable of doing that, but how would we learn? How would we grow? He's raising a mighty army, not a frail one. God allows affliction because it's the only way glory will be released. It's what increases our anointing. I've heard it said that you will know how anointed a person is by how much they've gone through. Your painful history gave you access to glory. Standing on this, don't ask God to remove the test. Ask Him to help you ace it. For this too shall pass, and glory will be your portion.

5. Show kindness. Kindness is the sugar that's sweeter than honey from a honeycomb, the activated grace that establishes your name.

- I find it comical how the fifth fruit also defines the spiritual term for the number five. That is, grace. Though we've touched on grace in a previous chapter, I need to magnify its description to help you fully understand kindness. The Greek word for grace is *charis*, which is the unmerited favor of God,[1] favor that is produced without works. I'm talking about the "I'll bless you just because," "I'll heal you just because," kind of favor. Ephesians 2:7 says the Father shows immeasurable riches of His grace in kindness toward us in the Messiah. His sacrificial heart is what gave Him a name on earth and in Heaven. His compassion produced a reputation.

Let's take a quick look at the Good Book.

On the road to heal Jarius's dying daughter, Jesus stops to give the woman with the issue of blood an identity. To the crowd, she was an unclean woman who bled for 12 years. People treated her as if she was a poisonous snake, as if they'd catch an illness if they were under the same roof as her. The disciples even dismissed her after she skated through the multitude to get to Jesus. This poor lady just needed help. She needed to be seen.

"If I could just touch His clothes, I will be healed," she mumbled to herself.

This woman had already exhausted her finances seeking medical relief. All she had left *was* her faith. Yet that was all she needed. God was moved with compassion when He felt the power transfer from His Spirit to her body. Her boldness caught His attention, and in return, He showed her the most attention she'd gotten in 12 years. He was the first Person to look past her issues and at her heart. The first Person to give her a name. He referred to her as His daughter. Here's the icing on the cake. She was the only female He independently addressed by that name as noted in Scripture. The woman who had the issue of blood became the woman saved by the Blood. *That's* an act of kindness.

This same compassion from God is recorded a few more times in the Word. He meets a leper, a man with swollen and crusty skin, who was also treated as an outcast. Jesus is filled with compassion, stretches out His hand, touches him, and washes him clean. (see Mark 1:41) *That's* an act of kindness. Five chapters later, He sees the 5,000 begging for wisdom and direction. The Bible says He's moved with compassion, because they are like sheep without a shepherd. They're hungry for more, so He feeds them both physical and spiritual food. *That's* an act of kindness.

Two chapters later, He sees the 4,000 begging again for wisdom and direction. He's moved with compassion. Then He blesses them with both physical and spiritual food. *That's* an act of kindness.

There's another occurrence where two blind men are hanging out on the side of the road, waiting to hear Him pass by. They ask for help, the people insist on shutting them up, but Jesus sees them. He has compassion and touches their eyes. Immediately, their eyes receive sight. *That's* an act of kindness.

In Luke, a widow loses her son. Being that it was her only son, she begins to weep over the coffin. The Lord sees her, He has compassion, then assures her it's in His hands now. He walks over and touches the open coffin. The young man, who was just dead a second ago, sits up and begins to speak. *That's* an act of kindness. (Luke 13-15)

If you notice, almost every one of those narratives show Jesus touching people who were seen as unclean, even down to the dead. He showed that kindness is displayed through a simple touch. This is what created His fame. By making Himself nothing, He honored people above Himself. When you genuinely empathize with others, hear their stories, desire to help, and be friendly, kindness gives you a name. It gives you a reputation. Remember what the Bible tells us. You'll know a person by the fruit that they bear. That's why the Cross is such a huge hit when the Bible is spoken about, because we remember Jesus for His kindness. He knew we would be in trouble, He had compassion on us, and He came to save us. That was the greatest act of kindness ever recorded in history.

Now, it's your turn to lead by example. Lend a hand. Lend an ear. When you open your heart in generosity, the warmth from people you touch will be empowering. "Give, and it will be given to you: good measure, pressed down, shaken together, and running over will be put into your bosom. For with the same measure that you use, it will be measured back to you." (Luke 6:38)

6. Do good works.

- Whereas kindness is grace-activated, the fruit of goodness is kindness-activated. The difference between the two is that fruit number five occurs as a reaction to a person or event. It's the compassionate butterflies that are felt when someone needs your comfort. This is why the examples I provided earlier involved Jesus reacting to the cries of His children. The sixth fruit is done on purpose for a purpose. Goodness is the intentional deeds of a kind-hearted person. A great example of this would be the "pay it forward" act.

  You're in the drive-thru at a fast food restaurant, like say Chick-Fil-A, and you reach the window to pay for your food. The attendant dismisses your money and tells you that the person in front of you took care of your tab. Instead of pocketing that money, you pay for the car behind you. This continues on until there's someone who really couldn't afford their order, and is able to keep that money for a rainy day. The first person to initiate the act did so out of the goodness of their heart. These are deeds that no one directly asked you for, but you willingly go out and find special avenues to uncover Holy Spirit.

  Other examples of goodness would be donating clothes, volunteering at a food bank, funding a charity, knocking on doors to pray for people, reading a book to disabled children, and singing at an elderly care facility.

Goodness is deeply honored by God. He chose us to be rich in good deeds and willing to share. In this, we'll line up treasure for ourselves as firm foundation for the coming age, so we may take hold of the life that truly is a life well-lived. (see 1 Timothy 6:18-19)

7. Stay faithful. Faithfulness is a divine marriage between you and Christ.

- In a wedding ceremony, the bride and groom are swept into a covenant: "I take you to be my partner, to have and to hold from this day forward, for better or for worse, for richer or for poorer, in sickness and in health, to love and to cherish, till death do us part." In discipleship, those same vows are appropriate, except death brings the opposite of division in such a case. Death pulls you closer to God. Dying to your emotions, your attitudes, your plans, and your ways, creates a marriage pact between you and Christ. There's a reason the bride walks down the aisle with her veil on and then removes it once she meets the groom at the altar. The veil symbolizes her will. Therefore, removing the veil shows that she is willing to give herself up for their new creation. The man and woman form as conjoined twins—sharing one mind, one body, one soul, one spirit, just as you do when you're born again.

    Upon entering life as a believer, you marry God. Isaiah notes that our husband is the Maker, whose name is the Lord of hosts. Call it holy matrimony if you will. This marriage stamps our names on His heart, and His on ours, meaning we cannot do what we wish. We cannot disown Him. We cannot doubt Him. We cannot grieve Him. We can, however, choose faithfulness. We can wait on Him. We can heed instruction. Let your waist be girded and your lamp burning, for blessed is she whom the Master will find watching by the door, waiting for Him to light a fire. (see Luke 12:35-48) Devotion takes the cake. Your life is not your own; it's the Lord's. You were designed by a jealous God. According to the second book, His name is Jealous. A definition for jealous is to be fiercely protective or vigilant of one's rights or possessions.[2] He's jealous because He's faithful to His possessions. He's faithful to His daughters as an earthly husband is to his wife.

You won't catch God cheating on us with another breed. His heart is always open for your desires, His kit is overflowing to meet your needs, and His schedule is forever free for intimacy. Knowing this, don't just date God whenever you feel up to it. Marry Him! Kiss Him! Stay faithful to Him! Do not let this be a one-sided relationship where the other Person is loyal and you commit adultery. Delete the tiny gods and make Him the head. Remove your veil and adopt His will.

8. Be gentle. Holy Spirit programs us to treat every human like a piece of glass, careful not to shatter their image or break their spirit.

- I ate this fruit the hard way when I began raising my own children. Gentleness choked me up at first. I come from a family with a mother who would knock your teeth out if you'd so much as think about going against her word. I'm a lot like my mom in that sense, but my crew is nothing like the age I was raised in. Self-entitlement, daring, and hardheaded are descriptions that befit my mini adults. Oh, how frazzled I get from repeating the same things to them in a day:

  "Josiah, quit jumping off the entertainment center. You are not a monkey." "Kaelyn, stop bossing your little brother around!" "Jo, quit beating up your sister!"

  Multiply these statements by 100,000, and you've got yourself a typical day in the Sparks's house. Although my kids are my joy, they're equally a pain in the butt. What parent do you know loves repeating the same things over and over again? What parent do you know loves being lied to? It's hard raising kids. They'll do jumping jacks on your nerves until you go berserk. Then you hate yourself when you consider the unholy exclamations that flew out of your mouth. This is where gentleness should be the prescription. Gentleness should be the toll we must pass before making a move, before we speak the first word.

The King wants us to be gentle, lowly in heart. Why gentle? Well, if you're not cautious, you'll fracture a person's identity. "X's and o's" would not work miracles for the sake of their future. I must be delicate with my children, as with all people, because I have the power to produce cancerous thoughts in a person's mind about themselves. Life and death are in the force of the tongue. Your words could blow someone's shot at self-love. Remember that phrase, *Sticks and stones may break my bones, but words will never hurt me*? Once upon a time that was taught to children as a weapon against bullying. I, myself, recall going around the elementary hallways and humming it after being mistreated. To my dismay, the stupid phrase was a lie. What my peers called me back then started to rip me apart in adulthood. Hello, Depression. Right?

No wonder idle words are mentioned in Matthew as those we'll have to answer for on judgment day. Idle speech is anti-God and serves no purpose. A gentle tongue, on the other hand, is pro-Spirit. Had Paul wrote the epistles with a bleep in every sentence, the Gospel would have a few kinks. People are not won over by hearing a list of wrongdoings. You win a person over by tallying up their high scores—being gentle with God's creation the way a mother is with her babies.

9. Stay in character. The fruit of self-restraint is having the power to improvise in the flame.

- I performed in a few plays in middle school, and I took drama class in high school. I absolutely loved entertainment. The chance to not be me, the center of attention, the costumes. I worshipped the theater. Aside from learning screenplays, one of my teachers would have us do warm-up sessions at the beginning of the period. These sessions were called improv. A group of us would be instructed to walk up to the front of the class and act without a written script. She'd give us nothing but a brief history of the characters and a plot to kick it off with. The dialogue and in-betweens were on us. This meant everything was fair game as long as we stayed in character.

  Like drama, self-restraint is all about staying in character. The Teacher provides the storyline: "Creation has fallen. I'm sending you into the world to fish for souls." He paints our character: "You'll be playing the role of the salt and the light." He emits the rules: "You may say or do whatever, as long as you respect My people."

  Perhaps the angel who appeared to Jesus in the garden of Gethsemane did not come to lessen the anguish. Perhaps he showed up to help Jesus stay in character. That would explain the gift He had to restrain Himself during the abuse. I find cases like this in the

Bible so enabling. If He did it, we can too. If the apostles did it, we will too. All we have to do is grab tips from the Word and act it out.

Scripture is our life jacket. Without it, mental seatbelts could never stay fastened. Brethren would have no filter. All nine fruits would decay. I reckon the absence of self-restraint is due to the self not allowing God to restrain it. How can Holy Ghost be our help, if we never let Him take the wheel? He's there to apply a divine coating over your flesh like a Snapchat filter to a picture. He smooths out the rough edges, split ends, and nasty pimples. He can prevent you from beating up the girl who called your banana rotten. He can remove the alcoholic taste from your mouth. He'll even run you out of the cookie aisle and direct you to the spinach to balance out your A1C. Don't misjudge this Powerhouse. He will not let you be tempted past your limits. Read the Menu of Life and learn the basics. Gain enough information to be able to improvise on eggshells.

Everything is fair game, as long as you don't let the character of another take you out of character. You are no longer acting out your own image. You have been selected to play the role of God. For we did not choose Him but He chose us and appointed us, so that we might go and bear fruit—fruit that will last—so that whatever we ask in His name, the Father will give us. (see John 15:16)

Part Two: His Ink is a Dose of Zinc

When you were designed, Father God needled His ink on you. You have a birthmark on your spirit. This mark came injected with a lifetime supply of zinc. Zinc is a nutrient found in the body which builds immunity and quickens metabolism. Zinc can also heal wounds and level your senses. This nutrient is accessible to you for the weary days when you run out of oxygen. Days that are clogged with gunk. Days when you cannot discern your right from your left. Days that make you wish there were life packs on the ground to give you an instant burst of energy and power.

Realize that you have been gifted with a life pack that can never be drained. Know that your birthmark is a super-suit. You have armor against destruction. Unlike the immune system, the Triune system is never-failing. He's your Ride or Die. Your Partner in Crime. The Solution to prevent you from growing weary in well-doing. There will be times when you're stretched so thin to the point where you just can't take anymore.

No more bad news

No more bills

No more awful relationships

No more persecution on the job

No more grief

This is what you use the ink for. This is when you call on God.

"Lord, I'm weak. My mind is weak. My heart is broken. This is as far as I can go on my own. Carry me on Your back, and help me see this through."

The forerunners of the Church had to cash in their ink for grit as well. In Acts chapter four, Peter and John were arrested for preaching the Resurrection. The Sadducees kept trying to shut them up by locking them up, but God sustained them. When they were stretched thin, the ink stepped in. They ignored the opposition and kept going forward, never looking back to see who had a problem with it, never stopping to complain about how hard it was. They found rest in the Lord as their Backbone, and He delivered them. On one occasion, an angel came and bailed them out. He opened the prison doors and told them to keep spreading the word. Their diligence in doing the right thing caused generations to be saved.

I, too, am familiar with being stretched thin. Do you recall the talks about my third pregnancy? By the end of it, Jace had my abdomen stretched so thin the skin became translucent and numb. I would poke at it with something sharp and couldn't feel a thing. My stomach was so prominent, people always had something slick to say about it.

"Hey, there's a good place up the mountain to give birth."

"Girl, I don't think that baby will make it through the night as big as you are."

"Goodness, are you 39 months pregnant?"

The comments hurt because they had no clue what was causing my bump to grow so large. Neither did they understand all of the physical pain I had gone through since week nine. I had to convince myself not to grow weary in well-doing. (2 Thessalonians 3:13) God wanted me to make this sacrifice to have a third child, and that's what I was doing. I was doing right by Him. I had to keep my head up. I had to keep running because I knew a harvest would come sooner than later. I knew the pain wouldn't last forever. I knew He would rescue me. That does not mean I didn't cry it out. I did! I cried. I became angry. I felt alone. But praying, and seeking, and knocking is how He strengthened my spirit.

To date, He's patching up my wounds and remolding my body. Things aren't perfect, but at least I have sensation in that area again! My nerves have reconnected! He's proven that if He broke it, He could mend it. If you're losing heart, He'll offer you His. If they persecute you, He'll release you. If He stretches you thin, His ink will step in.

Part Three: The Confessions of a Christ-like Obsession
How would you feel if you did surgery on a patient's brain for free and they denied it ever happened? The surgery was successful, and the OR team rejoiced with you. Your hands removed a tumor the patient had for 30 years. The only favor you asked of them is for your name to be mentioned. This favor was not on the basis of attracting popularity. It was on the basis of love. You desired to pull in sick people off the streets and heal them. Pro bono, at that. The patient couldn't take it upon herself to mention you because she felt that it was something you were supposed to do, as if you owed her the four years of medical school and seven years of residency you toiled for. She let you down, and it hurt. But that did not stop you.

You later find another person in need, perform an amazing

surgery, and they follow in the first patient's footsteps. The same process continues on until you finally stop and wonder why no one wanted to speak your name. That's all you were asking for. Has it ever occurred to you that Omega wonders the same thing? He heals, He delivers, and we stay silent about it, as if it's something He's supposed to do because He's God the Creator, as if He owes us. Humans aren't quick to say His name like we ought to be.

Honestly, it's like the Destiny's Child song.

"Say My Name" created a trend of women and young girls from all over, testing their man to see if he was cheating. Destiny's Child made us alert. If you suspect it, call him out on it. The only difference between the singing artists and *the* Artist was their motives. The song was written to catch the boyfriend in a lie. Jesus wants us to mention Him because, "Salvation is found in no one else, for there is no other name under heaven given to mankind by which we must be saved." (Acts 4:12) He wants us to be models of the Good News. He wants us to expand Heaven. One cannot be educated on the Good News if you never credit who's been good to you. Do you not want to see depression slayed? Do you not want to be the spokesperson for the Most High? Do you not want people to tell you that because of your testimony, they didn't give up? I do. Count me in. When you say His name, He'll make sure to run yours by the upper admin. Deny Him, and He'll deny He ever knew you. Don't get it twisted. He's not in debt with us. He works in our favor because we're His offspring.

There are three concepts I had to swallow when I began to grow my relationship with Christ:

1. He owes me nothing. Not a darn thing.
2. Whatever unfavorable situation I face is not an act of hatred. It's an act of love and leveling.
3. Every good and perfect gift in my life is not based on my merits. It's not because I followed every guideline in the Manual of Advocacy. It's here because Grace said I could have it. It's here because He put His name on it.

Humble your mind on this. Confess your journals about Christ. (see Matthew 10:32) Tell men, women, and children everywhere to hang onto the Word. Tell them there's more to life.

I was itching to expose the supernatural when He cleared my depression. I became obsessed with the Cross and wanted everyone to know what I'd been through. People asked if I would say His name when I told my story, or if I would sugar coat it with words like *the universe, forces of nature, the atmosphere.* I responded, "Why wouldn't I say it was God? My story could not be told without the Author. I'd be a fraud!"

I'm not ashamed. I'm activated. I didn't get here on my own. He drove me here. He marked me. He saved me. He chose me. I will forever say His name!

Therefore, although in Christ I could be bold and order you to do what's right, I prefer to appeal to you on the basis on love. (Philemon 1:8) So, here's an inquiry for you. When God heals you, are you going to scratch His name out? Or will you scream it from the mountaintop? I pray you won't get sidetracked by what others think of you. I pray you'll confess that you are Christ-like obsessed.

THE *Experience*

An **experience** is a sum of events, emotions, and knowledge (both past and present) that make up someone's character.[3] A woman can only live *for* God *as* God if she's had an experience with Him. An experience is what she'll remember when He seems distant. Short of one, she stands alone. She has no bone marrow, nothing to grab onto when attacks come knocking. A cell without a nucleus is what she becomes; only trace amounts of His DNA will be left over. The less DNA, the less structure. The less structure, the more pressure.

Part One: Unplug the Drugs

When a person suffers from breakouts on the skin, they purchase acne products to manage it. Sometimes, the best creams for acne will cause a purge of additional bumps to appear before the skin eventually clears. Dermatologists agree that skin purging is beneficial. The skin cell turnover rate speeds up, and it tacks off dead cells faster than normal. The final result? Healthy, younger-looking skin, free of blemishes, wrinkles, and uneven tone. You just have to survive the purge to see the gains.

When Heavenly Father visits our belly, He wants to purge. He wants to break us out before He clears us up. He wants to cut down into the epidermis and subcutaneous fat layers to remove any toxins, anything that causes you to lose sleep, feel low about yourself, or keep you from identifying holiness. He wants you to forge new memories, experience His fullness, tap out of society and into divinity. But before you tap into a God experience, you must first unplug. He once told me, "Adriel, you will only find Me when you're unplugged." To unplug is to disconnect a device by removing its plug from a socket. If your eyes, ears, and sense of touch are the sockets, then what you perceive in a day creates a plug for each—an emotional, physical, and mental connection to you.

The human shell was made to be highly receptive. Be highly selective on what it receives. Why? Because you're renting it out. It is not a mere body. It's the Lord's property. It's a temple for Him to find rest. Clean out His temple like you would if you were returning a car to Enterprise. Tidy up your sockets.

I'd like to unfold a physical temple as it relates to a human temple in order for you to understand how vital this is. Six parts make up a temple, the first of which is a double package.

1. **The doors and windows:** These are your gates of entry and exit. What are you letting in and out of your spirit? What kind of music do you listen to? Are the words encouraging? Do they heal your heart and mind? Do you find peace and harmony? Or are you vibing out to music that refers to women as hoes and -itches? Music that tells you it's perfectly fine to be self-consumed, clenched to a materialistic mindset, and hate everyone. Music that has no better topic than

drugs, sex, and money. What are you streaming on TV? Whose social media pages are you sliding through? Once you've given an honest reply to these questions, I want you to think about how strong of a bond your senses have to your spirit. Whatever you hear and see will give birth to your thoughts and actions. What goes in must come out.

2. **The floors:** On what grounds do you stand? Are you standing on the word of the Lord, or are you earthbound?

3. **The ceiling:** What is covering your head? What do you speak over your life?

4. **The altar:** What are you worshipping? Who's your master? Are you waking up every morning and checking your horoscope? Or are you asking God to prep you for stability? Are you fixated on calorie intake? Or are you reading a verse of the day? When you're down, do you turn to weed or to the Vine Himself? You could silently worship things and fail to notice it. Find out what those are and simplify them, for the Bible says you cannot serve two masters. You'll love one and hate the other.

5. **The pews:** What sits heavy on your heart day and night? What causes you to lose sleep, and is it worth it?

6. **The walls:** What boundaries do you have in place? If you know you have an issue with pornography, have you downloaded content blockers? If you spend too much time on your phone, have you tried limiting your

usage? If you always deplete your bank account, have you set up restrictions?

Do yourself a solid and unplug the drugs. The very health of your psyche depends on it. During your purge, ask yourself the "high five" to determine what you need to break away from.

1. Does this person or activity make you feel content?
2. Does your depression heighten or decline after its exposure?
3. Do you feel the urge to change who you are? (I'm not talking about the positive changes that God is making in you.)
4. Do you leave that person or activity feeling mentally drained or mentally full?
5. Does the Word support it?

If something you're tied to failed the *high five*, it may not be the healthiest for you. It's time to purge. Your mental health is far more important than a bad habit or fitting in. Start by saying "No." Titus 2:12 (NIV) says we have the right to say "No." We can unplug. We can tap out. No boxing match is worth losing focus on what's pure. Now, God will not make the switch for you if that's what you're waiting for. He's too much of a Gentleman. He does, however, shepherd you through it. But you must hear Him over them.

Cut the world off as much as possible until you learn how to discern. Stop watching so much of the news. It's drunken with useless info and keeps you anxious and topsy-turvy. If it's something you really need to know, God will find a way to get it to you. While you're at it, go on a social media hiatus for a bit. Two days out of the week. A month. Six months. Whatever feels right. I've done this twice now, and I feel completely free each time. The first one lasted approximately seven months. This second one I'm doing has lasted almost a year and a half. Media breaks are similar to a food fast. You starve the mind while being fed by Holy Spirit.

When you unplug the drugs, you plug into the goodness of God—giving Him a beautiful place to lie His head, prop His feet up, and relax in your temple.

Part Two: Silence Is Timeless

Silence. The complete absence of sound and the enemy of noise. For silence to function outside of time means there is no end to what you can experience. The silence will generate an unfailing, imperishable, and ageless meeting between you and Christ. This is the moment you launch your spiritual gifting. This is the moment you prove yourself to yourself. He knows who you are. Do you? I had no idea what He loaded in my vending machine until we met in solitude. After swiping the meditation card, all kinds of treats were released from me. In the silence is where I activated the gift of tongues. In the silence is where I found the prophetic. In the silence is where I discovered the seer anointing. Not in church. Not at a conference. Not in revival. He trained me in the supernatural from my living room. That's when I learned God was accessible anywhere, everywhere, and at all times. I don't have to wait until Sundays for Him to blow my mind. He can wow me 24/7!

Don't get me wrong here. Church is a great place to attend

when you've found a ministry you can call your family, though it's not the only place God moves. He moves in you first, then the people can have a piece of it. Can you imagine if this was flipped? It'd be like a football team playing in the Superbowl without practicing first. That's chaotic! God cannot use you until He first approves you. This is a training that's done in isolation, behind closed doors. He teaches you how to activate your gifts in today's silence, so you'll know how to share them in tomorrow's noise.

There are two levels of an experience: the sunken place and the takeover. The first level is the deepest form of meditation a person can enter. Sinking is like jumping off of a diving board and swimming to the bottom of a pool. The water hugs you. The distractions disappear. Your mind is clear. A vivid example of this is Jordan Peele's movie *Get Out*. Remember when Missy took Chris to the sunken place? She said one word, "Sink," and he fell through the floor. She hypnotized him by stirring tea in a cup and recalling a childhood memory. This is how deep the Father wants us to go. Into the sunken place. The God cave. No flesh allowed.

My number one tip for initiating the sink is to find a private area and meet God with a longing, a craving, some sort of a need. Begin your experience in worship or prayer, and give Him your undivided attention. Ask Him to let the rivers flow. Ask Him for a stirring. Ask Him to let His fire consume you. Then, sink. Fall into the Spirit. Let go and allow Him to take over. In the takeover phase, be still and know that He is God. Put on your virtual headset and create a new reality. Design a new experience. Make it a night to remember. Make it four dimensional if you can. Sometimes you'll sense Jesus so strong that it will feel like He entered the room with you. Get *there*. Desire *that* move of God.

Don't tense up when you find Him taking over. Ride it out. Go with it. Sure, it'll be awkward at first because you're no longer in charge. It's an experience you may have never felt, almost like reciting the ABCs in reverse. But He's got you. Close your mind and open your core. Allow Him to pour out His Spirit. Be filled with the Holy Ghost. Cry. Shout. Dance. Speak in tongues. Listen for His voice. Pay attention to what He shows you. Accept what your heart is beating to. And again, I say to you, be still and know that He is God. Be still and know that He is God. Be still. Know that He is God.

This is the hour He is awakening your spiritual gifting. Whether you're a prophet, a seer, a dreamer, a teacher, a pastor, an evangelist, a giver, an administrator, a healer, an interpreter of tongues, He will manifest them to you. "There are different kinds of gifts, but the same Spirit distributes them. There are different kinds of service, but the same Lord. There are different kinds of working, but in all of them and in everyone it is the same God at work." (1 Corinthians 12:4-7) The same Spirit. Just a different experience.

Part Three: Reproduce Your Juice

To reproduce is to re-birth your pro-duce. Produce is a section of the grocery store that houses fruits and veggies. Out of the two, fruit is the only food that contains seed, making it the only life-bearing food. If He is the Tree, you are the fruit. If you are the fruit, you hold the seed, seed that carries new life. A fresh anointing. Oil in a cup. What are you to do with it? Drink it all by yourself? Eat by yourself?

No, actually. You have to set it free. You must give birth to that seed. God reproduced us so we can reproduce. It's the gift that keeps on giving. The blessed that keeps on blessing. The led that keeps on leading. You ever heard the phrase, *To be sure you know a topic, go out and teach it*? Well, I'll do you one better. Now that you've activated the fruit basket, go out and juice it, pulp and all. What good is it for Kingdom if you just sit on God's wisdom? Anyone who runs ahead and does not continue in the teaching of Christ does not have Him. Whoever continues in the teaching has both the Father and the Son. (2 John 1:9) That woman is a firstfruit. She's a bearer of the Word. A leader of the blind and the brokenhearted. You have it so you can spend it. How do you spend it? By teaching the ropes of activation.

Take a sister to the School of the Holy Spirit and train her from the Textbook. Be the inspiration. Get involved with the reproduction of the House. Spread the Word through your gifts of ministry, your hobbies, your career, your friendships. Think outside the box. Instead of just having pizza with a friend, make it a "pizza and purpose" night and talk about identity. Produce photocopies of your light and have fun with it. Write it. Speak it. Sing it. Show it. But no matter what you do, preach it. Preaching it will help you stay fired up for God and focused on the prize. Help your sisters overcome what you're working on yourself. Fix each other's crowns. Elevate, encourage, and empower. Search for ways to hold yourselves accountable in this healing season. Breathe Scripture over one another. It has the power to teach, rebuke, correct, and train in righteousness, so the woman of God may be thoroughly equipped for every good work from here on out. (see 2 Timothy 3:16)

You are the product of reproduction. Go and reproduce your juice.

THE
Dividend

A **dividend** is a benefit that arises from an action or a policy.[4] It's the advantages, the bonuses, the extras, the perks of being activated as the Word. 2 Peter 1:3 (NIV) writes, "His divine power has given us everything we need for a godly life through our knowledge of Him who called us by His own glory and goodness." The dividend is your divine end. Your final destination. A multi-level stairway to Heaven.

The First Flight: Calculus on Cannabis

I've been in love with mathematics since the fourth grade. I remember having an assignment on the multiplication chart where the teacher gave us one week to learn numbers one through twelve. I went home and studied that chart with everything in me. I repeated those numbers incessantly until they became engrained:

$5 \times 2 = 10$; $8 \times 8 = 64$; $3 \times 7 = 21$.

My motivation was to hear a job well done, "You did it, Adriel, and I'm proud of you. Here's an A+." I did not expect anything more than a good grade and a pat on the back. That was plenty for me. When test day rolled around, I came in the class pumped, ready to ace that thing. I put up my bag and sat down at the desk. The teacher handed out the multiplication sheet, and I went to work on it:

6x8 is 48. 5x12 is 60. 3x8 is 24.

Grades came back the following day. Turning the sheet over with a hopeful look on my face, I saw that I had not only earned that A+, but I became the new *Student of the Month*. I was the only one in the class who knew every single multiple by heart. She rewarded me with twice as much as I hoped, and it blew me away.

This is precisely how God operates. He works in the spirit of multiplication, where simple digits turn into the dividend. He takes your "A" and maximizes it. What you've lost, He multiplies it. What you haven't labored for, He opens up the door. It's a type of calculus that creates a high like cannabis.

Cannabis, as you know, is the plant responsible for marijuana. It contains two famous cannabinoids: THC and CBD. CBD is non-euphoric, meaning it doesn't get you high. Instead, it relaxes you. THC, on the other end, can harvest elation. THC is what I like to call **"The Holy Calculator"** because the favor of God is an incalculable high, one that your brain is unable to process. It's beyond the beyond. You don't know a high until you've experienced that. How would I know? Well, I've gotten high in the past, and I hated it. Weed did nothing but leave me with a horrible taste in my mouth. Getting high in the Spirit? Now that's euphoria. Good fortune that makes your head twirl. Still need reassurance? Let's go back to the book of Amos in The Message Bible: "Yes indeed, it won't be long now." God's decree. "Things are going to happen so fast your head will swim, one thing fast on the heels of the other. You won't be able to keep up. Everything will be happening at once—and everywhere you look, blessings! Blessings like wine pouring off the mountains and hills. I'll make everything right again for my people." (Amos 9:13-15 MSG) These verses paint calculus on overdrive. To better grip this thought, however, we need to redefine this term.

Calculus, which was formerly named infinitesimal calculus, is a branch of mathematics that is concerned with instantaneous rates of change and the summation of infinite factors.[5] God, being the Infinite Father that He is, multiplies our blessings at instantaneous rates of change. God's math is limitless and makes no sense. He took five loaves of bread and two fish and multiplied it to feed 5,000 men, then collected 12 extra baskets of leftovers! That's five times two equals 5,000, carry the 12. That's not regular math. That's calculus on cannabis. Then He took seven loaves and a few fish and multiplied it to feed 4,000 men. The disciples collected seven baskets of leftovers at the end. That's seven times a few equals 4,000, carry the seven. That's not regular math. That's calculus on cannabis.

The same spirit of multiplication is shown in Job's story as well. He starts off a righteous and wealthy man who owns 7,000 sheep, 3,000 camels, 500 yoke of oxen, and 500 female donkeys.

Job loses everything: his employees, his 10 children, and the health of his body. At the end of the story, though, God gives it all back plus bonuses. He multiplies his property and leaves Job with 14,000 sheep, 6,000 camels, 1,000 yoke of oxen, 1,000 female donkeys, and 10 more children. Job lives out the full of his days and is able watch four generations give birth to his name. That's not regular math. That's calculus on cannabis. If favor did not function this way, humans would have a reason to gloat. We'd have faith in ourselves and wouldn't need God. So, to avoid this, He more than doubles what we ask.

I had a vision about the spirit of multiplication one day. In the vision, I saw the Lord fishing at a lake. He would throw the fishing rod into the water, catch a fish, and throw it off to the side in a boat. He continued until the fish became so big that He had to physically take His hand and grab them out of the water. The fish began to transform into a beautiful mix of iridescent colors. They were hues of purples, blues, and gold. Once the boat was nearly full, He turned around and said to me, "These could be your blessings if you follow Me." I later saw Him grab the largest fish and drench it in oil as He spoke the words, "I pour My anointing on them," and He threw that one off into the boat of blessings.

This same spirit of multiplication is being offered to you right now. All He needs is your obedience. He wants to take you into unseen realms that are going to substantiate the Word that lives in you. He's even said that His people would do greater works than He. That's saying a mouth full! If He, the Living God, demonstrated so much power during His time that the world itself is too small to keep record of, how much more do you think He's willing to do through you? Eyes have not seen, and ears have not heard the things that the Lord will multiply for those who love Him.

All I can say is buckle up because you're in for the Uber drive of your life.

Second Flight: The Beginning of a New Ending

I titled this section based off of it being a step up from *Calculus on Cannabis*, but not quite Heaven yet. It's more like Heaven on earth. He wants to give us a slice of the pie right now before we spend eternity with Him. Unlike Santa Claus, who can only work Christmas miracles on one night, the Creator works Christmas miracles by the minute. It's the millions added to your $40,000 salary. It's the nine-level jump from your assistant's position. The CEO status at one of the largest companies in the world. The piece of art in a museum that sells for 3 times as much as you originally priced it. The book that takes you from living in your car to buying a penthouse in upstate New York. The online business that allows you to quit your well-paying job. The website that acquires more traffic than Amazon. The audition that relocates you and your family to Hollywood. The struggling associates degree that sets you up to receive your PhD. The 400 credit score that shoots to an 850. The clothing company a celebrity advertises for. The food truck that expands into 100 restaurants around the world.

The opportunities are boundless when the Lord marks you. He pulls you to the side and says, "Aw, that's cute. But that's not enough. Watch Me amplify this." He graciously gives into those who hold His name. He cordially presents you as His joy. He knows what you want and just how to provide it. He's got everything in His Designer's bag. God never runs dry of magic. He pulls off the impossible at any given moment, as many times as He wants, for as many as He wills. That's Elohim. The only True and Living God. He gives, and gives, and gives until we break into tears. Then He give us more just in case we thought He was finished. The gifts never stop flowing, and the miracles knock us down when we least expect it. This is Heaven on earth. But it's only the beginning of a brand new ending.

Third Flight: Life in Paradise

"Enter by the narrow gate; for wide is the gate and broad is the road that leads to destruction, and many enter through it. But small is the gate and narrow is the road that leads to life, and only a few find it." (Matthew 7:13-14 NIV) I wanted to include this last stage prior to the birth, so you'd have something to hold on to when dealing with transition, to let you know the difficulties you've faced were worth it.

A mother goes through a lot during pregnancy. She gets to a point when she just wants to quit. She's tired of the swelling, the heartburn, the sleepless nights. As a means of keeping herself encouraged, she'll try to stay reminded of how happy she'll be when she gets to hold her baby, when their eyes connect in admiration, as if she's entered a new life in paradise.

Like her, you've been through a lengthy course as well. You've successfully completed all nine months of pregnancy.

You've accepted Christ as your Lord and Savior. You've allowed Him to come in and eat with you. He's been your Professor at the University of Life. You've revisited your old birth certificate. You've acquired new vision, new access, new character, and new experiences. You've done it all. The Trinity has made Their home in you. But now, God wants to give you a baby shower gift, the greatest advantage of all. The perk above all perks. He wants to let you know that no matter what happens from this day forward, He has prepared a place for you. A place that can only nurture serenity and bliss. A place where there are no more tears, sorrow, anguish, or depression. A place where you will no longer have to fight for your life. Somewhere for you to finally rest your soul. A place to commune with the Word of God face to face, shoulder to shoulder, hand in hand. A forever with the Forever. An eternal get-together with the Alpha.

Meet Paradise.

The final home for the activated. The final dwelling for the woman of God. The Holy City. The Throne Room. The Divine Estate. The Peace Palace. The Narrow Way. The Promised Land. And as you've heard it said, the Third Heaven.

ACT *on this!*

Godly character is a major part of identity. The word "identity" means to ID the entity on which you build your footing. Any woman who desires to be more like Jesus has to let go of her own image and identify herself as the Word of God. In order to save a soul, you have to play the role. Christ tells us that the earth would know His people by the fruit they bear. As believers, we must bear love, joy, peace, patience, kindness, goodness, faithfulness, gentleness, and self-control in our everyday lives. In agreement with God, what are some ways you can juice the fruits of the Spirit in your personal life and career?

NINE KEYS TO THE DOOR OF

activation

1. Get to know the holy basics.
(The Arrival)

2. Build a three-part relationship with Christ. (The Confidant)

3. Swallow chunks of spiritual wisdom. (The Teacher)

4. Reclaim your name.
(The Identity)

5. Plant your purpose.
(The Vision)

6. Unlock the Blood Bank.
(The Access)

7. Trade your mark for His.
(The Trademark)

8. Tap out of society, and into divinity. (The Experience)

9. Blow kisses to depression, and fall in love with Heaven.
(The Dividend)

WHEN YOU HEAR THE
VOICES RISING AGAINST YOU,
BATTLE THEM WITH THE
WORD OF GOD

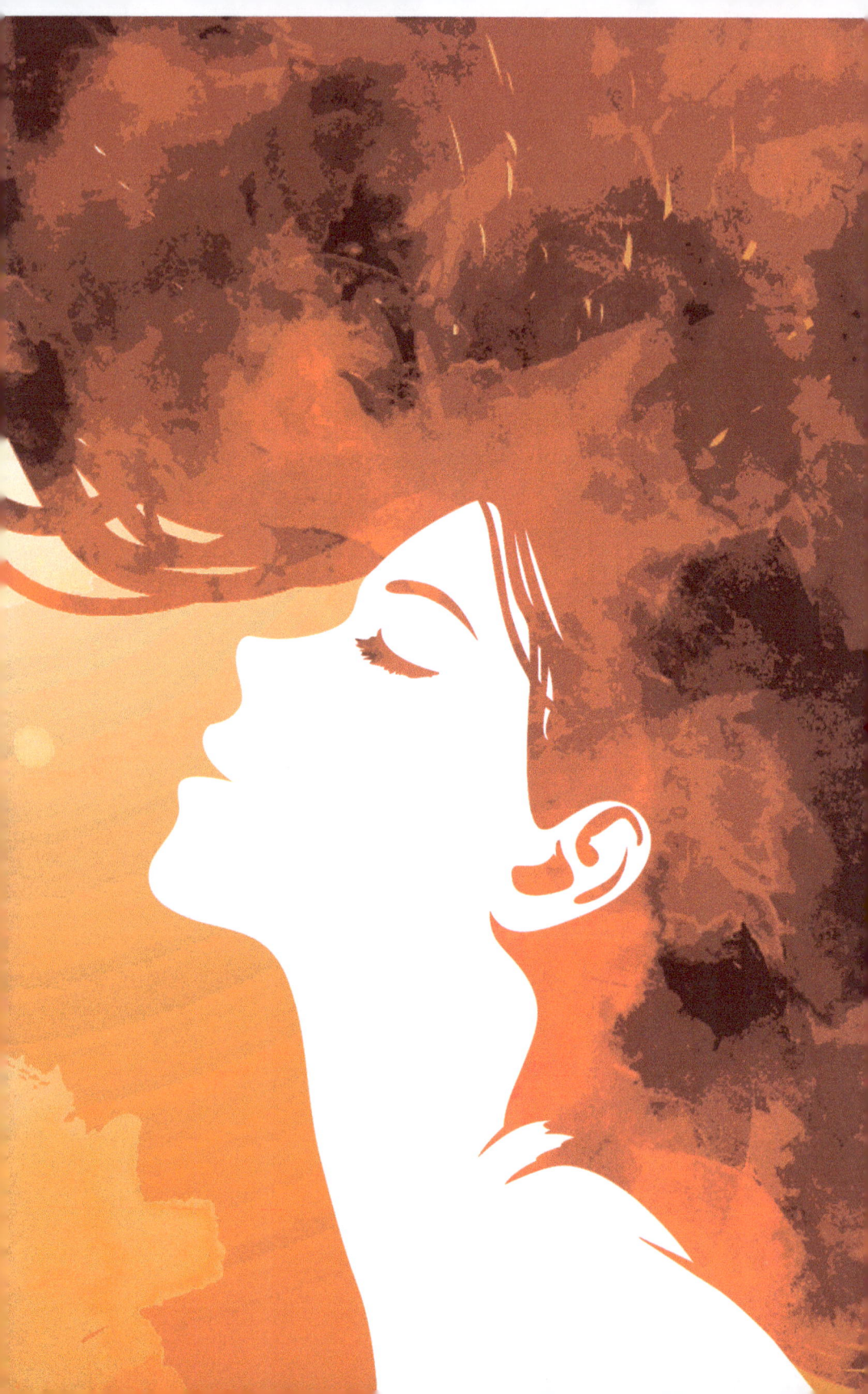

CHAPTER NINE

BIRTH OF THE WORD

Your water has broken, and you're rushed to Labor and Delivery. The nurses check you in and attach your hospital bands. The patient ID reads: 333. You change into your glory gown and lie down on the bed. You're about three centimeters dilated, and contractions are two to three minutes apart. It's time to have a baby!

THE CONTRACTING PHASE
trust the process

"Okay, deep breaths. Try your hardest to relax. Listen to your body and go with the flow. Trust the process. You're doing great, Mama."

This is what you hear midwives, obstetricians, nurses, and family members telling the woman in labor who chose the unmedicated route. Like it's so easy to let your body expand farther than its resting state—accompanied by the shooting pains that make you want to punch your husband in the face. Natural childbirth is no joke. It's the nearest thing to death they say, and I agree. I thought I was going to die when I birthed my first son unmedicated. I turned into the exorcist. In fact, I'm sure I was the loudest patient on the floor that day. It was dreadful. Your body is ripped apart during birth to deliver that human's head through your vagina. The cramping is like your period on crack. Your patience wears out. Your pain level reaches a trillion on a scale of one to 10. You are ready to have that baby. You want your body back, your emotions back, your sex life with hubby back. I've been there three times, and it sucks.

Contractions are like HIIT exercises, high-intensity interval training. Runners who participate in this type of training alternate between rapid sprints and light jogging. They repeat that same process for miles at a time or until they're exhausted. That's pretty similar to the rhythm of contractions. Your cervix draws up into the body of your uterus, and your walls start to thin until it's safe for baby to exit. The contractions last about 30 to 70 seconds each, and the intensity builds as labor progresses. It's normal to tense up when you feel a contraction coming on because you're afraid of the impending doom, the pain that you've felt before. The pain you now know so well.

This is rebirth. Getting delivered is no walk in the park. It took a lot of stress and disappointment to bring you here, and it's going to take a lot for you to fully cleanse. Do not be alarmed if you're stuck with the repercussions for a few months. There will be times when you feel like the Enemy is still in control. Suicide may even stop by to check on you. Whatever you do, go with the flow. Trust that you are being healed. I contracted a few times after my jumpstart to freedom. Depression went away and left anxiety to have its last-minute fun. I'd have many days of pure bliss with the Lord, and out of nowhere, fear would attack me. My nerves would send me into those familiar panic attacks. Except this time around, I had trouble finding the trigger point. The attacks went on for a few months before I figured out what caused them. Anxiety would appear after I engaged in "Mommy" duties, conversations with people, and large crowds.

When you go from being numb all the time to feeling normal emotions again, you're delicate. It's like healing a broken toe. Though it functions much better after being coddled, you get jumpy. You're cautious about the injury. You find yourself moving out of the way of other people's feet, standing off from the edges of couches, and carefully turning corners. You don't wish for a thing to set back your healing. Believe me, I would know. I'm suffering from a sprained toe as I'm writing this, and the heat wave of a person scares me. It's similar to how I felt when I wrestled against the demons in my mind.

I journeyed into the wilderness to find the light, but anxiety and depression would try and prevent me from escaping. There were objects that I had to climb over and throw to the side to make it out alive. The gnashing of teeth and animal howling made the hair on my arms rise. The fear was orchestrated by Satan to keep me in his war hole.

This time though, I could feel it. I could feel the contractions of the Word birthing through me. I could feel my identity reaching. I could hear my purpose calling my name. So, I gave in to it. I gave into the activation, and I trusted the process.

Even with the negative thoughts racing in my mind, I told myself, "I trust it." Even with the family members who failed to understand my battle, I said to myself, "I trust it." Even with my heart beating out of my stomach in the middle of a conversation, I told myself, "I trust it." I knew I would get through it.

The same God who saved me from multiple suicide attempts is the same God who will hold my hand through psychological labor. He was doing something on the inside that was bigger than a few setbacks. The purpose in my belly was larger than life. Not only was He delivering me, He was using my testimony.

I had to get through it for you. I had to write this story. I had to choose life to give you the same opportunity. Just like me, you have to make a choice for her—the other woman who will need your testimony. Birthing as the Word will be your greatest victory, but no birth comes without pain. It does, however, welcome a reward.

God Himself had to labor through contractions. There's a reason He didn't come here as a grown man. He needed to be born again to teach us how to rebirth. He wanted to show us how to trust this phase. How to win the game. The temptations He faced were beyond what we experience today. We're talking about the entire world on one Man's back. Though He knew there was an army of angels who could save Him from death, He trusted the plan. He chose us instead of Himself, and in the end, the Father gave Him what He'd promised. His pain was only temporary. His purpose? That was everlasting.

Take it from Jesus. Contractions will be painful, but they're only temporary. Trust the process. You can do all things because He covers you. "For every *word* of God is flawless; He is a shield to those who take refuge in Him." (Proverbs 30:5)

You are a flawless word of God. Owing to that, He has you guarded. His strategies to help you through labor are crisp, refined, and dished on a plate of good order.

THE RING OF FIRE
trickery of the enemy

You're not worthy enough to come to God for help.

He won't hear your prayers.

Your sin is too deep to be forgiven.

You will never make it out alive.

Depression will torture you forever.

Anxiety will always be your closest companion.

You don't know who you are aside from mental illness.

You'll never live up to your calling.

What makes you think you're good enough?

If I were you, I'd curse the day I was born.

If I were you, I'd curse God for what I'd been through.

No one will ever love you.

You'll always feel small in a room full of people.

You'll never see prosperity.

You'll never really find your purpose.

Just quit while you're behind.

Kill yourself already; you're wasting space on Earth.

Oh, the joys of hearing the serpent's voice haunting you as you're still fighting your way to freedom. This is when the contracting phase is taken up to the maximum level of discomfort. Say hello to the ring of fire, the most painful stage of childbirth, therefore making it the most painful part of activation. This is when you've reached your peak of self-doubt, and you may feel a suicidal attempt beginning to surface. This is the crossroad between the devil's world of terror and the Light of Life. The Enemy sees that you're stepping foot into the heavenly abode, and he seeks to destroy you one last time before you enter.

After hearing the word over my life and clinging to my promise, his tricks deceived me. A rude comment made by a man in Walmart threw me over the edge when I got back into the car with my husband. Wyll didn't understand why I had gotten upset over something so small. I tried to explain it to him, but we argued. We went back and forth the entire ride. I became so overwhelmed that I opened the car door and tried to jump out. I was sick of being misunderstood, and I couldn't figure out why I was still fighting Goliath.

I can't do it. I'm not strong enough. I'm still mentally ill.

These thoughts circled my head as I slowly circled the drain.

I began to scream out loud, "I don't know why You chose me, God! I can't get through this!"

Then He calmly said to me, "Because you *will* get through it."

After I heard Him speak, I had a decision to make. I could sink into a grave, or I could use God as an escape. Guess what, I chose Him.

I responded to my thoughts differently this time. I began to pray in the Spirit. There weren't any positive words for me to speak in English, so I preached the Word of the Lord to myself. I spoke in tongues the entire ride home, with tears flowing down my face and snot running from my nose. I prayed until peace took over. That was the moment I knew I was going to be okay. God would see me through the fire. I had discovered a rapid cure, and it worked.

Satan's plot was to make me doubt my activation and crawl into a dark space like I had always done. To his surprise, I fought against it, and I won. Again. I fed on God's medicine. With His medicine, came my victory. With my victory, came my serenity. With my serenity, came my healing. With my healing, came my identity. I'm the chosen one. The ring of fire burned me, but the furnace purified me. I'm a crystal formed out of magma. I'm a diamond fashioned under pressure. I'm a ruby molded from heat. I'm the Father's treasure piece!

It is the fire that makes a woman invaluable. It is her Lord who coaches her through it. When you hear the voices rising against you, battle them with the Word of God. Satan tempted Christ in the wilderness, and He responded with Scripture. The devil had no choice but to leave. If you don't know how to speak in tongues, that's okay! I've already taught you that there's power in the Verses. The Bible says that if we just speak a word, we shall be healed. Scripture is alive and active. It's sharper than any double-edged sword. It penetrates even to dividing soul and spirit, joints and marrow. (see Hebrews 4:12) Remember that the Word is your cure because you're word-activated! At the name of the Lord, every knee shall bow. Including Satan's!

When the devil says to you, "You're not worthy to come to God," remind him of this:

"The Lord will both help and deliver me because I trust in Him." (see

Psalm 37:40)

When he says, "The Lord won't hear your prayers," say this:
"This is the confidence I have in approaching God: that if I ask
anything according to His will, He hears me. And since I know that
He is listening—whatever I ask—I have already received." (see John
5:14-15)

When you hear, "Your sin is too deep to be forgiven," tell
him this:
"He has removed my sins as far away from me as the east is from the
west. He is like a Father to me, tender and sympathetic." (see Psalm
103:10-14)

When the serpent says, "You will never make it out alive,"
say this:
"The Lord will guide me continually and satisfy my desire in scorched
places and make my bones strong; and I shall be like a watered
garden, like a spring of water, whose waters do not fall." (see Isaiah
58:11)

When he says, "Depression will torture you forever," say
this:
"For I consider that the sufferings of this present time are not worth
comparing with the glory that is to be revealed in me." (see Romans
8:18)
"And even though I walk through the valley of the shadow of death,

I will fear no evil, for God is with me; His rod and staff will comfort me." (see Psalm 23:4)

When the Enemy says, "Anxiety is your best friend," say this:
"The peace of God, which surpasses all understanding, will guard my heart and my mind in Christ Jesus." (see Philippians 4:7)

When the devil says, "You don't know who you are aside from mental illness," say these affirmations:
"I am fearfully and wonderfully made." (see Psalm 139:14)
"I am God's temple." (see 1 Corinthians 3:16)
"I am royalty." (see 1 Peter 2:9)
"I am a new creation." (see 2 Corinthians 5:17)
"I am a crown of beauty." (see Isaiah 62:3-5)
"I am a daughter of the King." (see Romans 8:14)

When he says, "You'll never live up to your calling," place this on your heart:
"I am His workmanship, created in Christ Jesus for good works, which God prepared beforehand, that I may walk in them." (see Ephesians 2:10)
"For those God foreknew He also predestined to be conformed to the image of His Son, that she might be the firstborn among many brothers and sisters. And those He predestined, He also called; those He called, He also justified; those He justified, He also glorified." (see Romans 8:29-30)
"…nothing that I propose to do will be impossible for me." (see

Genesis 11:6)

When Satan asks, "What makes you think you're good enough?" say this:

"I did not choose Him, but He chose me and appointed me that I should go and bear fruit, and that my fruit should abide, so that whatever I ask the Father in His name, He may give it to me." (see John 15:16)

"The power of the Holy Spirit has come upon me, and I am a witness to the ends of the earth." (see Acts 1:8)

When the spirit of death says, "If I were you, I'd curse the day I was born," respond in this manner:

"I was born for such a time as this." (see Esther 4:14)

"He who created me...He who formed me...I fear not, for it is He who has redeemed me, and called me by name. I am His." (see Isaiah 43:1)

"Before He formed me in the womb He knew me, and before I was born He consecrated me; He appointed me a prophet to the nations." (see Jeremiah 1:5)

When darkness says, "If I were you, I'd curse God for what I'd been through," state this:

"For He knows the plans He has for me, plans to prosper me and not to harm me, plans to give me hope and a future." (see Jeremiah 29:11)

"Christ who died for me—more than that, who was raised to life

to give me life—is at the right hand of God, and will always be interceding for me." (see Romans 8:34)

When you hear, "No one will ever love you," say this:

"For I am sure that neither death nor life, nor angels nor rulers, nor things present nor things to come, nor powers, nor height nor depth, nor anything else in all creation, will be able to separate me from the love of God in Christ Jesus our Lord." (see Romans 8:38-39)

When the devil says, "You'll always be the lowest tier," respond with this:

"I am like a living stone, being built up as a spiritual house, to be a holy priesthood." (see 1 Peter 2:5)

"For many are called, but few are chosen. I, myself, have been chosen." (see Matthew 22:14)

When he says to you, "You'll never be wealthy," preach this:

"When I take delight in the Lord, He gives me my heart's desire." (see Psalm 37:4)

"He will supply my every need according to His riches in glory in Christ Jesus." (see Philippians 4:19)

When the devil says, "You'll never truly find your purpose," say this:

"I will seek first the kingdom of God and His righteousness, and all these things will be added to me." (see Matthew 6:33)

When he says, "Quit while you're behind," state this:

"Do you not know that in a race all the runners run, but only one gets the prize? I will run in such a way as to get the prize." (1 Corinthians 9:24)

"God is faithful; He will not let me be tempted beyond what I can bear. But when I am tempted, He will also provide a way out so that I can endure it." (1 Corinthians 10:13)

"As for me, I will be strong and will not give up, for my work will be rewarded." (2 Chronicles 15:7)

When you hear, "Kill yourself already, you're wasting space on Earth," scream this at him:

"I am the salt of the earth and the light of the world. I will let my light shine before others, that they may see my good deeds and glorify my Father in heaven." (Matthew 5:13-14)

Because Satan loves to come against you, make sure to put him in his place—beneath your feet. There is nothing he can say or do that will break you. He is the insubordinate angel who fell like lightning from the heavens. His lies are officially cancelled. God has given you the power over him. Use it to your advantage. I don't care if you feel the tiniest hint of God's presence or spoken word welling up in your heart, call out to Him with the crumbs you have left! Cry out His name when you just don't know what else to say. He has the first aid kit that'll resuscitate you on the spot. Use your "heavenmergencies" when you're injured.

You will labor through this. Just keep on breathing, Mama.

THE DELIVERY

Weighing in at 1,000 pounds of glory and 800 ounces of purpose, you have become a new creature. You are a powerful woman who has been fruitfully activated as the Word of God. You know what it feels like to thrust into the bottom of a rock. You also know what it feels like to have access to *the* Rock. The tough resistance that you've faced has caused you to doubt who you are, but the holy hormones have upgraded you. You have surpassed the limits of breakthrough. I'm proud to call you my anointed sister and friend. The Lord is overjoyed to name you His seasoned heir. He's held your hand during the pregnancy with Him, and He'll keep you under His wing during the birth as Him. Never forget that Holy Spirit is with you. With Him, you have everything you need.

He's the Knower of all things.

The Depression Dynamite

The Anxiety Axman

The Serpent Crusher

The Universal Ingredient

The All-Around Life Guru

There is nothing you cannot achieve with God on your side. No road too wide, no mountain too tall. The world's access card has been granted to you, and every entryway is word-activated. Watch as you enter the gates of triumph with facial recognition. Watch Him increase your favor. All will feel the presence of God when you step into a room now. Your name is on glory's guestlist.

That said, leave the past behind you. Past failures and regrets mean nothing from this day forward. God could care less about it because He's done a new thing. 2 Corinthians writes, "If anyone is in Christ, the new creation has come: The old has gone, the new is here." What does this mean? It means let it go! Whatever happened in your past has no effect on your calling. When God saves, He takes care of the whole timeline. He's the Beginning *and* the End. Nothing you did yesterday affects you today.

Hypercritical believers tend to forget this little detail. We have been wrongfully taught that our past banishes us from the face of God. Some are even told that mental illness is a result of sin. None of this is true! He calls for the broken—those of us who have jars of tears and burning thorns in our flesh. We are the pioneers. Christ is not a mean jock looking to bully you into doing the right thing. He's a patient, loving, and kind Father looking to save you. He's on the hunt for your heart. That's it: to make you feel comfortable enough to enter His bed and breakfast with your luggage of pain.

The war is over now, and you're ready to exit the furnace. Your body has bronzed, your eyes have flamed, and your hair has whitened as snow. You look like the Word of God. Your chapter of becoming has ended, for you have now become. You have become a strong woman of faith and force. You are a double-edged sword. The fight in the womb was trying, but the life outside was worth every speck of your death. This day, I declare everything be made anew. A new beginning, a new order, a new creation, a new you.

There will be no more "less thans" or "not enoughs." No

more delays. No more hiccups. No more confusion of self. You will no longer equate with the chewing gum stuck underneath the table. Nor the dead racoon that was slain in the middle of the road. We've suited you for a beautiful set of wings. We've placed diamonds in your crown. We've stamped your forehead with the Trademark. So, arise and celebrate your kingdom makeover.

The journey is now. Like wine, you've been harvested, crushed, fermented, clarified, and wrapped for marketing. He chose you out of the grapevine, crushed you to break off the limits, improved your makeup, sterilized your outpour, and labeled you as His fine ingredient in the end.

As the saying goes *the older the wine, the better it tastes*, the more you've lost, the more you have to give. Your pain has made you appetizing.

Mark today's date. For at this moment, it is done. You have won. So, fly high, Love. Go create something. Dance your heart out. Move somewhere you've always wanted to live, and don't look back. Become what you've always wanted to be, and don't spoil the renovations. Whatever pulls on you to grow, go with it. Whatever pulls on you to fall, leave it to die. He's calling you toward success. He's calling you toward fulfillment. Projects, businesses, and discoveries need you. We are waiting for you to be revealed.

Make yourself known. Shower God's globe with ambition. Remember His blessing over you: "Be fruitful and increase in number; fill the earth and subdue it. Rule over the fish in the sea and the birds in the sky and over every living thing that moves on the ground." (Genesis 1:28) Occupy the universe. Continue to sprout. Let your rose petals flourish. Sanction the sun to rise again. Let the ocean rest in your gut. Be pleased by the glistening dust running from your fingers. Admire the grace in your footsteps.

The things that have been spoken should give you peace. In the world you *will* have tribulation, but be of good cheer, He has overcome the world. (see John 16:33) You lost it all just to find it all in Him, and now you've found more than what you initially bargained for. You have found your truest road of activation. The Pages of Life have been dialyzed into your blood. You are empowered from head to toe, inside and out—physically, mentally, and spiritually. You've trained for this. You've even broken a couple of bones for this. But you've been granted the world championship belt, nevertheless.

You are…

THE ACTIVATED WORD.

ACT
on this!

I really hope this book has been
a blessing to you. What plans do
you have for yourself after reading
it? Have any new goals or ideas
kindled your spirit? Have any prior
ambitions been activated again?
If so, I am overjoyed, and I pray your
strength in the Lord. If not, don't
be discouraged. I can assure you that
when you give your life to God, He
manifests His glory through you. All
things will work together for your
good when you seek Him first.

"

DO NOT PUSH PRAYER

TO THE BACK OF THE BUS.

ALLOW IT TO BE YOUR

GAS PEDAL.

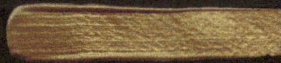

Prayers of Genesis

ACTIVATE GOD'S HEALING
POWER THROUGH PRAYER

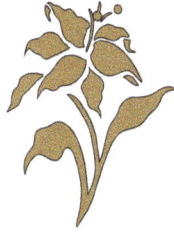

a genesis is an origin of a thing. It's the source, the root, the beginning, the evolution, the birth, the creation—the shaping of a person, place, or purpose. Genesis is also the first book of the Bible, which highlights God's power to write a masterpiece out of nothingness, the book that shows us how to activate a vision with words. Because the remedy to depression is centered around making you a new creation, I've generated a seven-day prayer list according to the Creation Week in Genesis. Notice that Saturday ends the week; it is the true Sabbath day. Luke 23 tells us that Jesus died on Preparation day, which is now called Good Friday; the women rested on the Sabbath, which was a Saturday; and He rose that Sunday. So, from Sunday to Saturday, I want you to inject these prayers in your spirit. Use them to help activate your days in addition to the healing methods drawn throughout this book. They'll mend your heart and strengthen your mind. Do not push prayer to the back of the bus. Allow it to be your gas pedal.

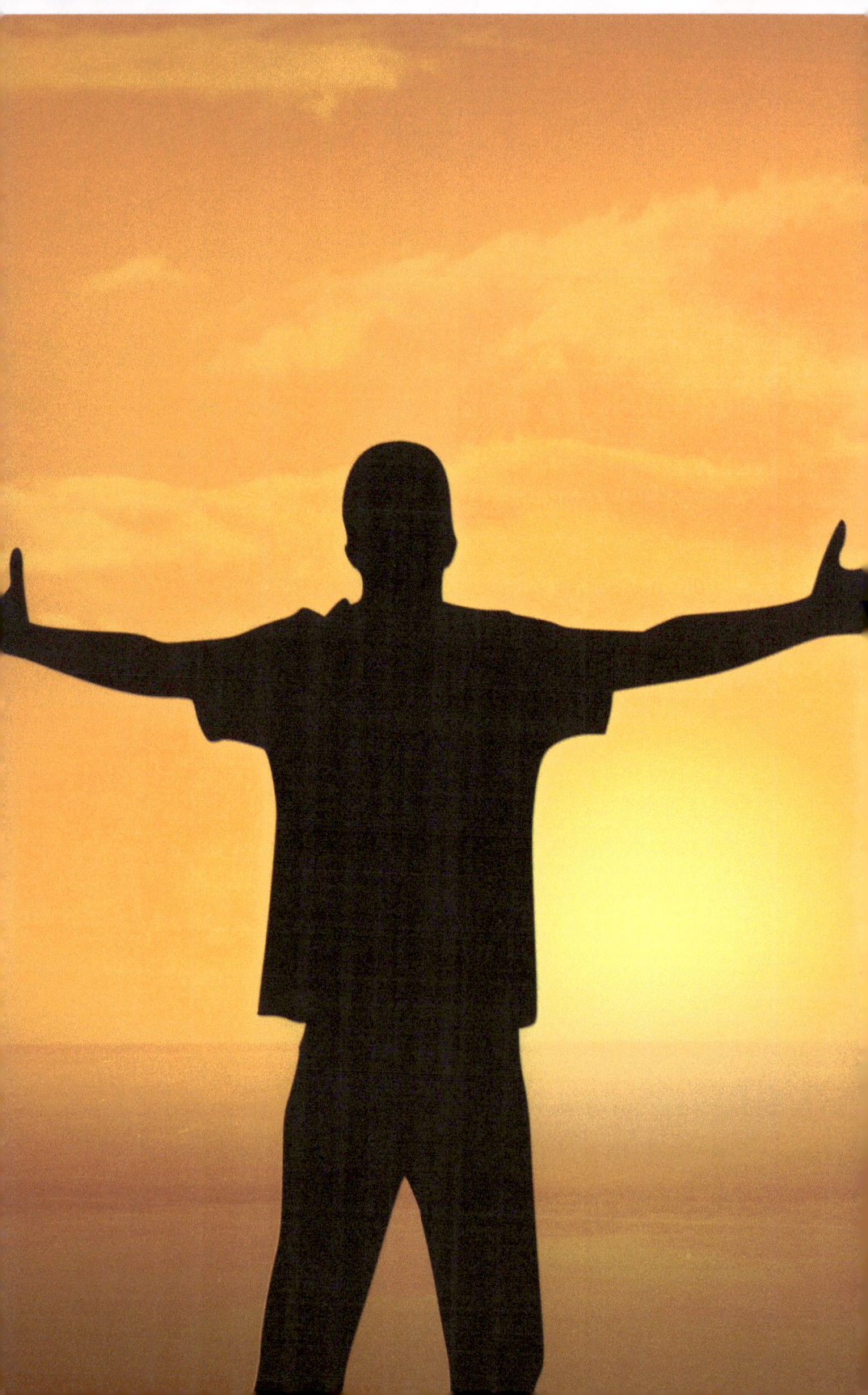

Sunday

On Sunday, God created light out of darkness, He divided the light from the darkness, then identified light as "day" and darkness as "night." There was evening and morning the very first day. (Genesis 1:3-5)

Pray this with me:

"Heavenly Father, this is the day You made all things new. This is the day You called light from nothing and raised Christ from the dead by the same glory. I ask that You illuminate Your Spirit in me. Create joy out of all poor situations that may come my way. Push me to divide the Enemy's speech over my life by reminding me of my roots in You. Continue to unfold my identity as one of the chosen generation, a royal priesthood, a holy nation, and Your own special possession, that I may proclaim the praises of Him who called me out of darkness into His marvelous light. In Your name I pray, Amen."

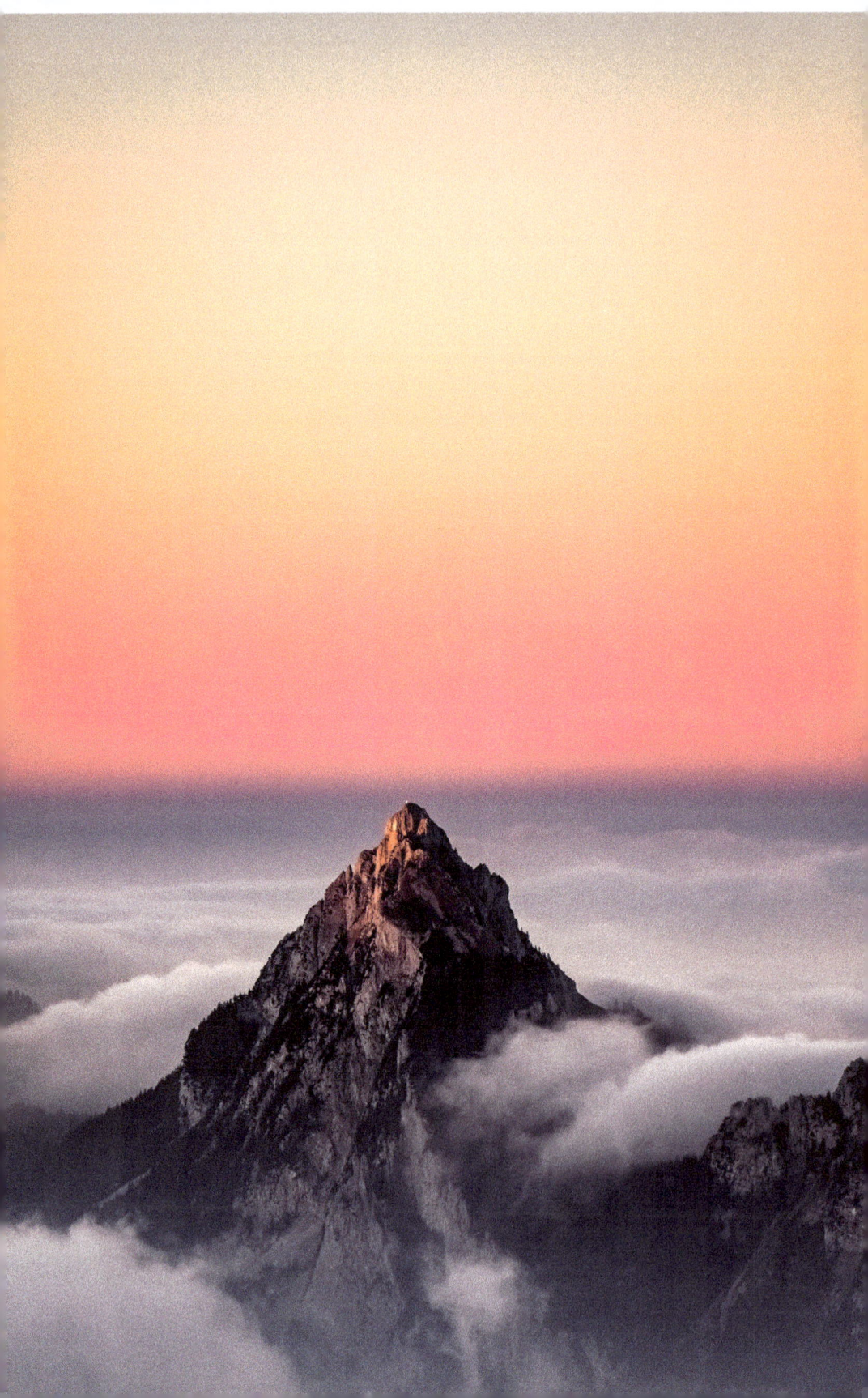

Monday

On Monday, the Lord created a vault to separate water from water. He stationed water above and below the vault and named the vault "sky." There was evening and morning the second day. (Genesis 1:6-8)

Pray this with me:

"Lord, on this day there was a prophetic separation of the waters. The water above represents Your will. The water below represents my own. Today, I ask that You give me one cup to drink from. One will. One authority. One mind. One heart. One vision. In Christ. Let me taste the everlasting well of life that You offer free of charge. Bring me to a place where I can't see anything but You. A place where I only crave You. In all my ways, I submit to You today. I have faith that You will make my paths straight.
In Jesus' name I pray, Amen."

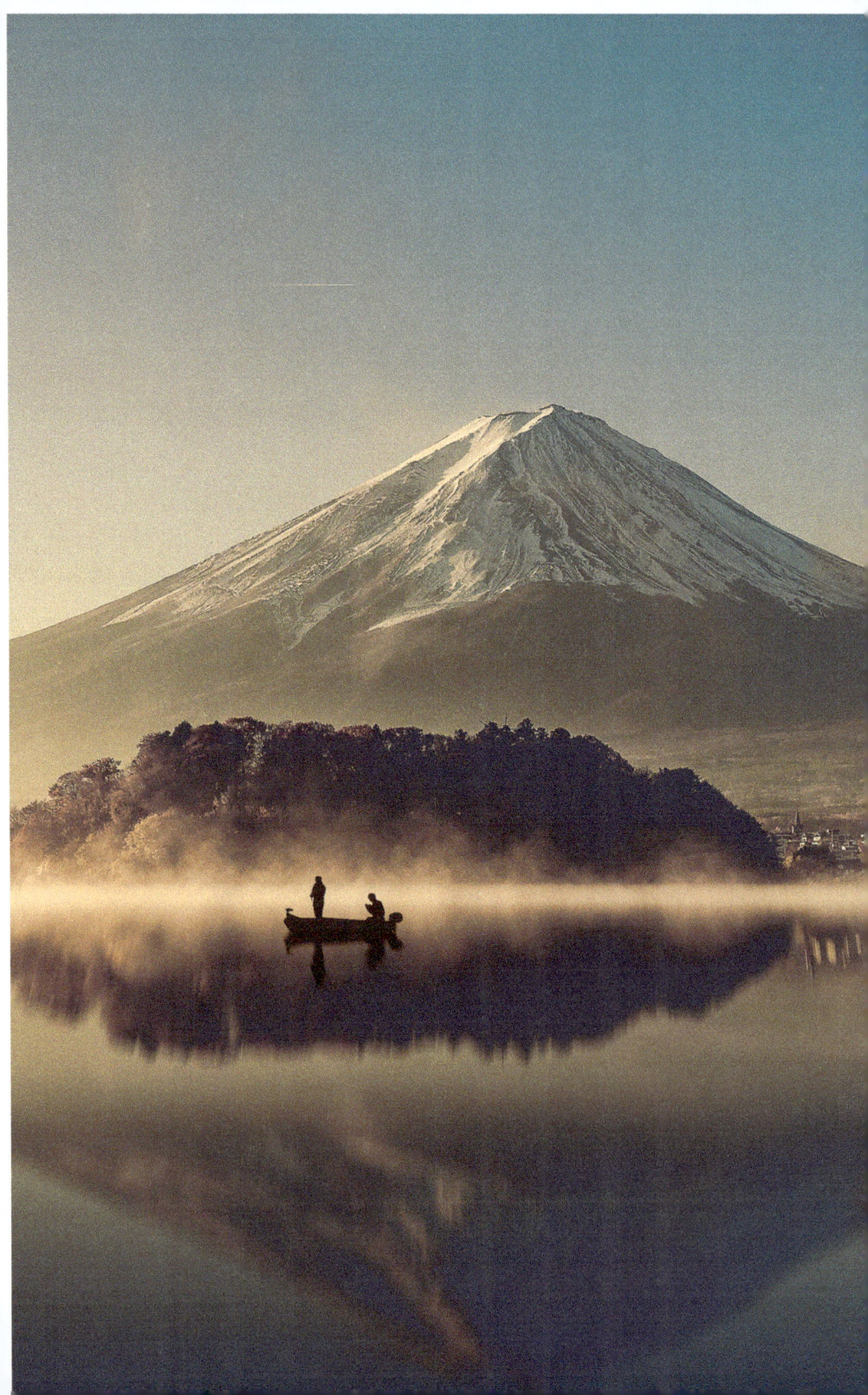

Tuesday

On Tuesday, the Lord created seas, land, and vegetation. There was evening and morning the third day.

(Genesis 1:9-13)

Pray this with me:

"Holy Father, as salt brings flavor to the sea and I bring flavor to the land, I pray that You bless the fruit of my womb. You are the True Vine, and I am the branch. Cut off what has spoiled in my life and prune that which has honored You. Season my gifting. Add grace to every good thing that holds my name. Allow me to not only see financial wealth, but a richer anointing—character prosperity. Build this temple on solid ground and remain in me as I remain in You, for I know that I can do nothing by my own efforts. In Your name, Amen."

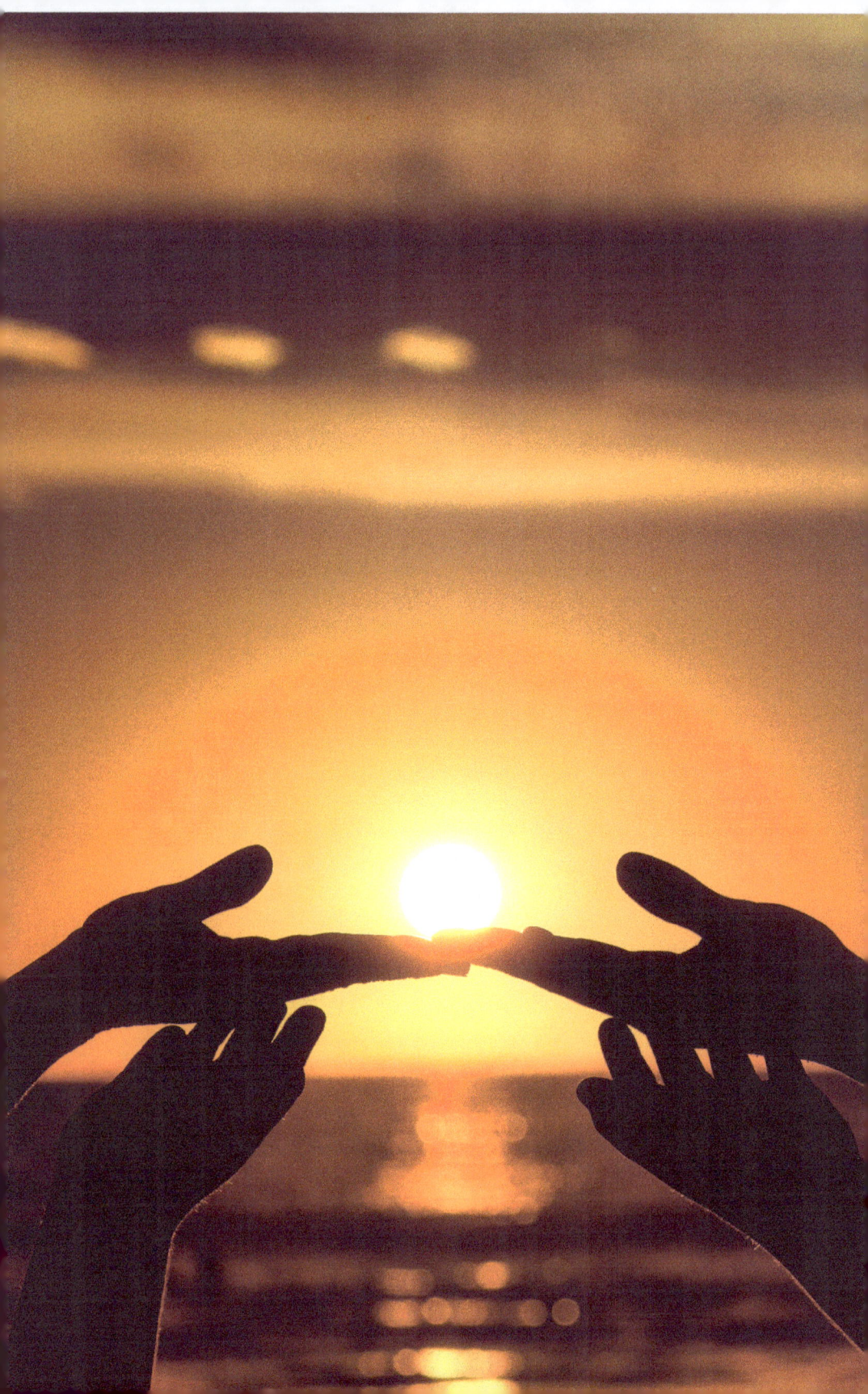

Wednesday

On Wednesday, the Lord created two bulbs of light. The greater light, which rules over the day, became our sun. The lesser light, which rules the night, became our moon. Then He adorned the night sky with stars too many to count. These final touches of His canvas were made to mark sacred times, days, and years. There was evening and morning the fourth day. (Genesis 1:14-19)

Pray this with me:

"Lord, mark my days with Your Breath. Allow the Word to multiply in my heart like the diamonds in the sky. Place Your flaming hand on my belly and let me sense Your power racing through my veins. Fill me with an angelic blaze that tears up strongholds. Set me on fire with God-intention. Let my spirit burn hotter than the UV rays from the sun. Activate my calling to such a degree that people will touch the hem of my garment and be saved. In Your name I pray, Amen."

Thursday

On Thursday, the Lord made birds and sea animals.
There was evening and morning the fifth day.
(Genesis 1:20-23)

Pray this with me:

"Father, it is written that she who waits on You will renew her strength. She will mount up with wings like eagles. She will run and not be weary. She will walk and not faint. So today, God, I will wait until You say 'go.' I will heed instruction. I will unplug disturbance and tune in to Heaven. You are the Shephard, and I am Your sheep. Comfort me with Your rod and staff. Help me to imitate Holy Spirit's guidance like the mockingbird. Make Your voice near and my hearing clear. In this, I declare strength is mine. Tough skin, thoughts of steel, and a bullet-proof shield. In the mighty name of Jesus, Amen."

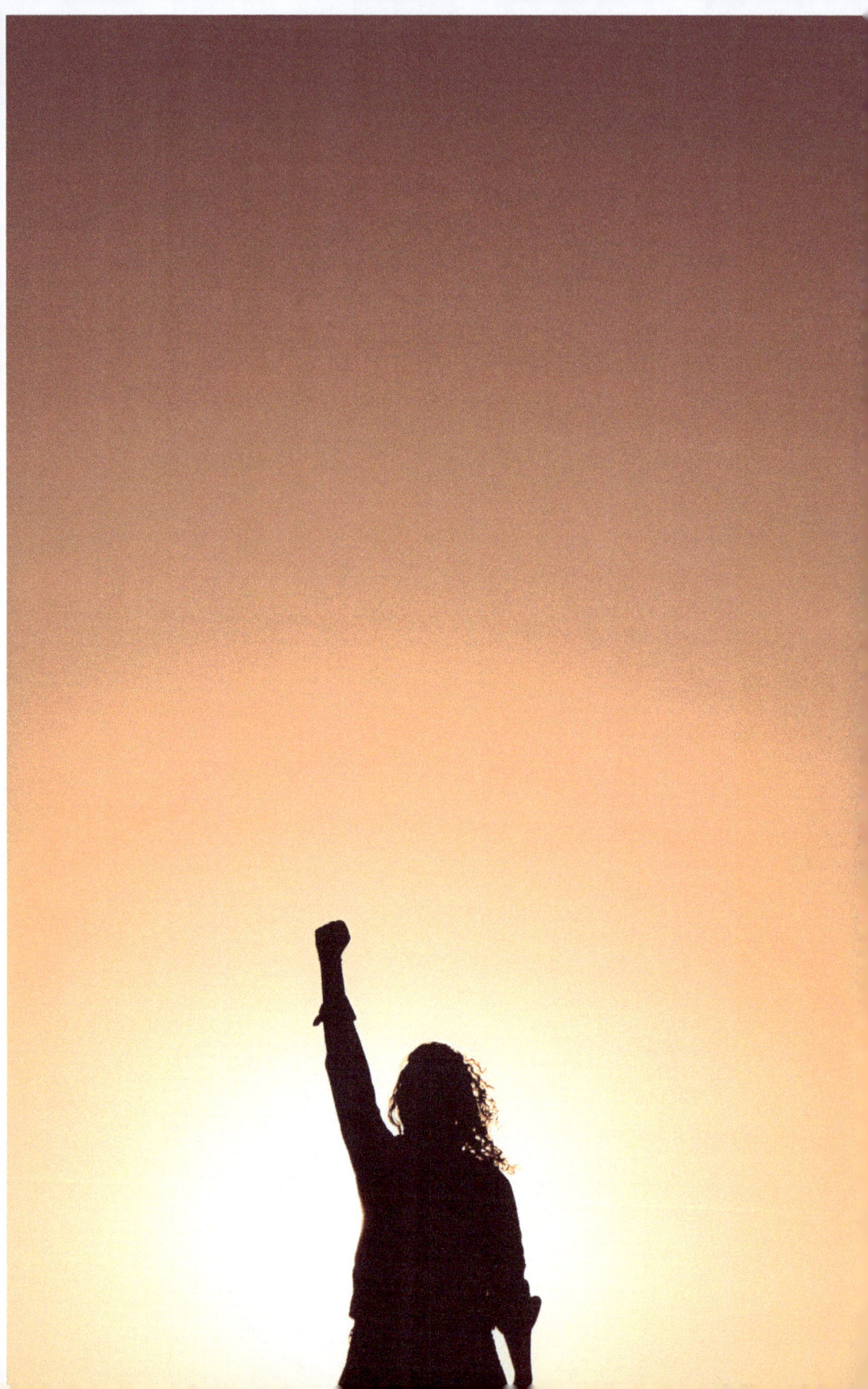

Friday

On Friday, the Lord created you in His likeness. He also added land animals in the mix. There was evening and morning on day six. (Genesis 1:24-31)

Pray this with me:

"God, I love how there are no coincidences with You. Every piece of Your artwork is fashioned into one stunning puzzle. I see it as no mistake that Friday is the day You chose to create man and die on a cross for us. The invention and reinvention happened on the same day as planned, and excellence was the result. There are no mishaps with You. There are no mistakes. A completely perfect God is incapable of imperfection. Being made aware of this, I thank You that I am not a mistake. I thank You that my birth was not by accident. You created me on purpose for a purpose, and for that I magnify You. For that I will die to the flesh and walk by the Spirit. In Your precious name, Amen."

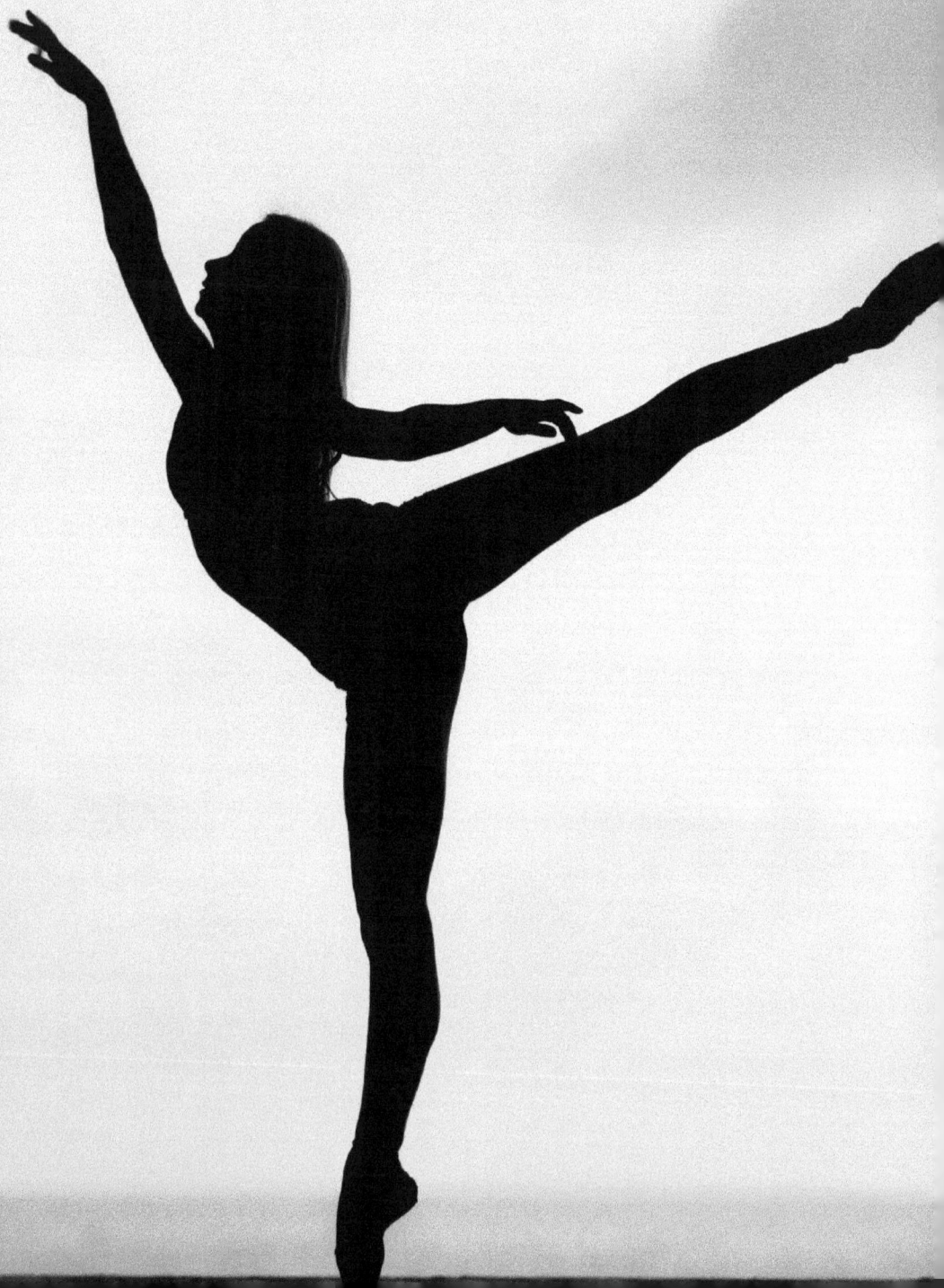

Saturday

On Saturday, the Lord rested and He blessed it. He blessed this day and made it holy. (Genesis 2:2-3)

Pray this with me:

"Lord, I speak total restoration over my mind today. A full turnaround. Peace without limits. Glitch-free serenity. Patch up my wounds and fly me far from past hurt and failure. Shut the door on mental skeletons that target my calling; those that are after my fortune. Lock out every bit of doubt and hopelessness that tell me I'm not worthy because I know very well that You have made me worth it. Today, I will rest my head on Your chest and feel Your heartbeat, as I am confident that You can heal the blind, cure cancer, and still have enough time to spend with me. Your fathership is a blessing all on its own, and Your intimacy is addicting. Thank You for being the purest form of love I could have ever asked for. In Your holy name I pray, Amen."

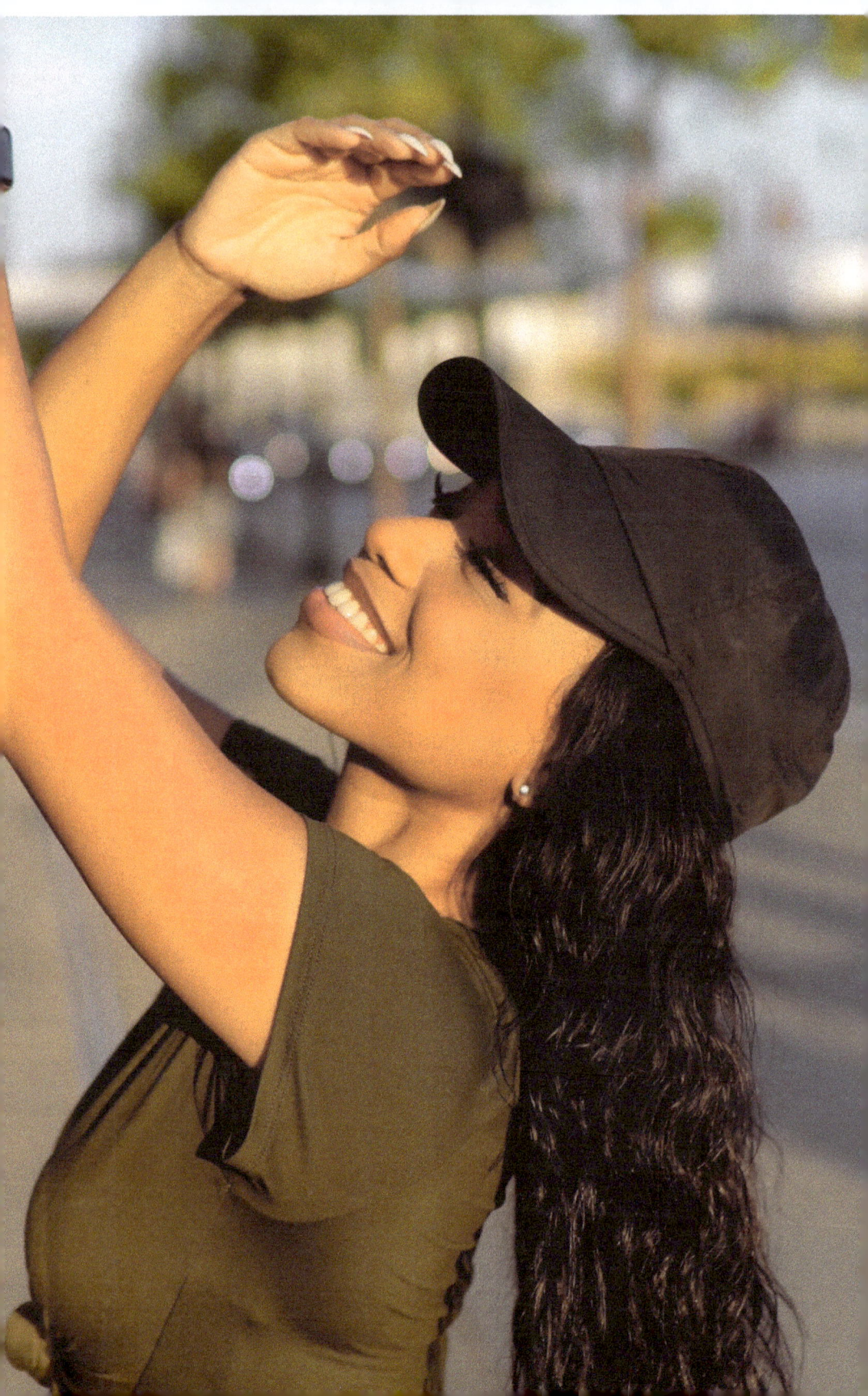

Meet the Author

ADRIEL NICOLE SPARKS

A wife to a faithful husband of nine years, a mother to three beautiful children, and a creative writer and graphic designer for her ministry's power-packed newsletters, call her determined. Adriel is passionate about spreading God's love and helping women find their truest identity. As someone once damaged by childhood abuse and many forms of mental illness, she believes your destiny is birthed from resilience. Her message is: *"You'll never discover who you are until you've been molded under the pressure of a fire."*

WHEN YOU'RE NOT

fasting...

📷 ADRIELNICOLESPARKS

🐦 ADRIELNSPARKS

f ADRIELNICOLESPARKS

👻 ADRIEL.NICOLE

📱 SCAN ME

my website!

What has this book
done for your heart?
Whatever that may be,
I'd love to read an
Amazon review
about it!

TELL ME YOUR

thoughts.

notes

CHAPTER 1

1. "Where Does Food Waste Go In The End?". Toogoodtogo.Org, 2021, https://toogoodtogo.org/en/movement/knowledge/where-does-food-waste-go-in-the-end.

2. New Oxford American Dictionary (Second Edition)

3. American Psychiatric Association. Diagnostic and Statistical Manual of Mental Disorders (DSM-5), Fifth edition. 2013.

4. Wisner, Katherine L., et al. "Onset Timing, Thoughts of Self-Harm, and Diagnoses in Postpartum Women With Screen-Positive Depression Findings." JAMA Psychiatry, vol. 70, no. 5, 2013, p. 490. Crossref, doi:10.1001/jamapsychiatry.2013.87.

5. "Depression." World Health Organization, 2020.

6. "Does Social Media Cause Depression?" | Child Mind Institute, 2021.

7. "Suicide Statistics." World Health Organization, 2016.

8. Laura A. Pratt, Ph.D, et al. "Products October 2011." Centers for Disease Control and Prevention, Oct. 2011.

9. Andrews, Paul. "Things Your Doctor Should Tell You About Antidepressants." Mad In America, 2 Sept. 2015.

CHAPTER 2

1. Department of Justice, Office of Justice Programs, Bureau of Justice Statistics, National Crime Victimization Survey, 2018.

2. "Approved Child Abuse Identification Course - New York State Mandated - Access Continuing Education, 2021.

CHAPTER 4

1. Mjl. "What Is the Meaning of Chai?" My Jewish Learning, 2 Nov. 2017.

2. Nelson, Thomas, et al. The NKJV, Woman's Study Bible, Hardcover, Red Letter, Full-Color Edition: Receiving God's Truth for Balance, Hope, and Transformation. Revised, Thomas Nelson, 2017.

CHAPTER 5

1. Ross, Hugh. The Creator and the Cosmos: How the Latest Scientific Discoveries Reveal God. 4th ed., RTB Press, 2018.

2. "Word Root: Con | Membean." 2017.

3. "Ception Meaning ." Your Dictionary. Accessed 2021.

4. "DISCOVERING HU." ORDER OF MELCHIZEDEK, atam.org/DiscoveringHU.html. Accessed 2021.

5. New Oxford American Dictionary (Second Edition)

6. "Recursion Meaning ." Your Dictionary. Accessed 2021.

7. New Oxford American Dictionary (Second Edition)

8. Amos 9:13-15 MSG

9. New Oxford American Dictionary (Second Edition)

10. New Oxford American Dictionary (Second Edition)

CHAPTER 6

1. "-ER (Suffix) Definition and Synonyms | Macmillan Dictionary." Macmillan Dictionary. Accessed 2021.

2. Klein, Bill. "PROSEUCHOMAI* - Greek Thoughts- Language Studies." StudyLight.Org, www.studylight.org/language-studies/greek-thoughts.html?article=147. Accessed 2021.

CHAPTER 7

1. Diamond, Dan. "Just 8% Of People Achieve Their New Year's Resolutions. Here's How They Do It.". Forbes, 2021.

2. New Oxford American Dictionary (Second Edition)

3. New Oxford American Dictionary (Second Edition)

4. Cherry, Kendra. "Comparing the Amount of Neurons in Human and Different Animal Brains." Verywell Mind, 10 Apr. 2020, www.verywellmind.com/how-many-neurons-are-in-the-brain-2794889.

CHAPTER 8

1. "Greek Lexicon Entry for Charis." "The NAS New Testament Greek Lexicon." 1999.

2. New Oxford American Dictionary (Second Edition)

3. "Experience." The Merriam-Webster.Com Dictionary, www.merriam-webster.com/dictionary/experience. Accessed 2021.

4. New Oxford American Dictionary (Second Edition)

5. Berggren, John. "Calculus | Definition & Facts." Encyclopedia Britannica, www.britannica.com/science/calculus-mathematics. Accessed 2021.

You are more gifted than you know,
more beautiful than you see yourself as,
and way more anointed than you feel.
Take the world by storm, woman of
God. If He's for you, no one can
be against you—not even you.

-A

Your takeaways.

_____

_____

_____

_____

_____

_____

_____

_____

_____

_____

_____

_____

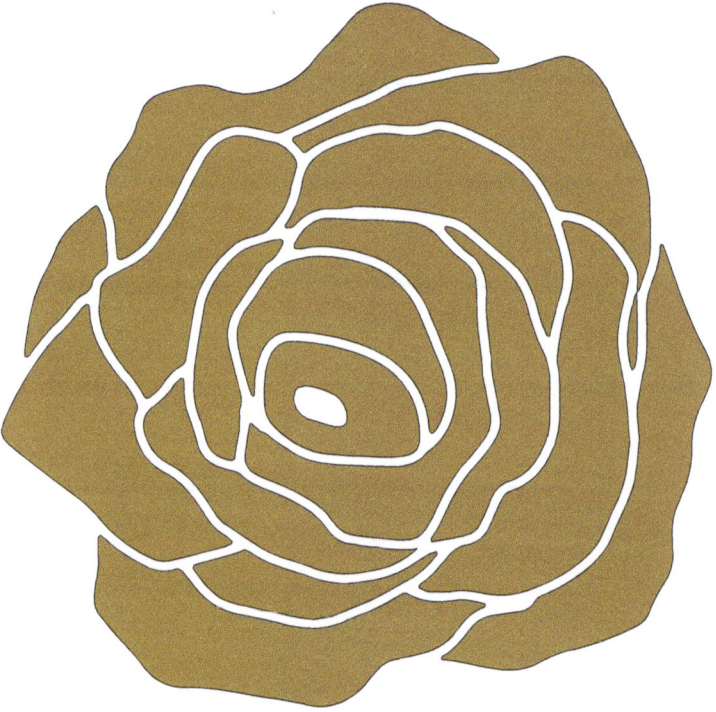